TOUCHED BY NATURE

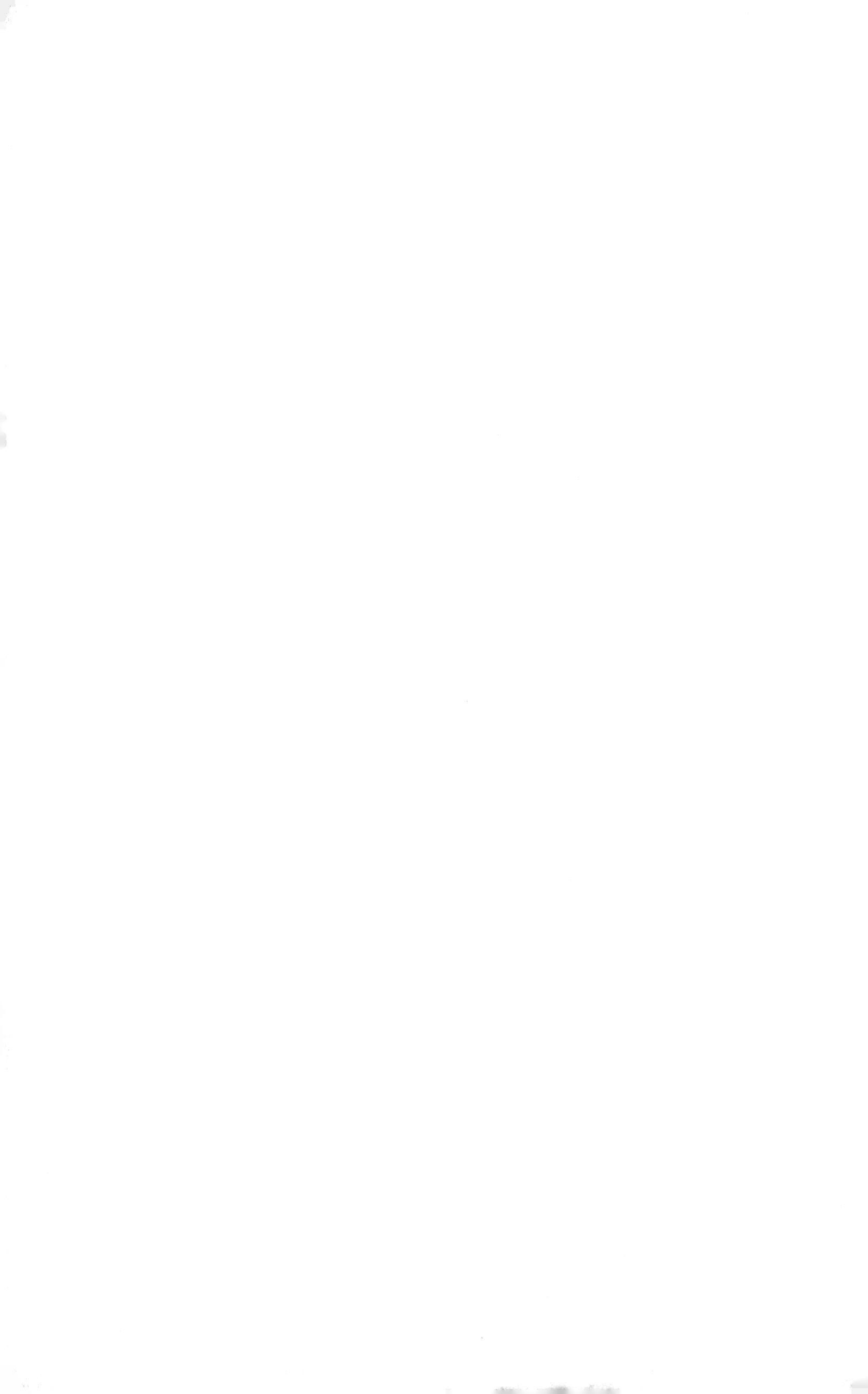

TOUCHED BY NATURE
Plant Spirit Medicine Journeys

Pip Waller and Lucy Wells

AEON

First published in 2019 by
Aeon Books Ltd
12 New College Parade
Finchley Road
London NW3 5EP

Copyright © 2019 by Pip Waller and Lucy Wells

The right of Pip Waller and Lucy Wells to be identified as the author of this work has been asserted in accordance with §§ 77 and 78 of the Copyright Design and Patents Act 1988.

All rights reserved. No part of this publication may be reproduced, stored in a retrieval system, or transmitted, in any form or by any means, electronic, mechanical, photocopying, recording, or otherwise, without the prior written permission of the publisher.

British Library Cataloguing in Publication Data

A C.I.P. for this book is available from the British Library

ISBN-13: 978-1-91159-763-6

Typeset by Medlar Publishing Solutions Pvt Ltd, India
Printed in Great Britain by TJ International Ltd, Padstow, Cornwall

www.aeonbooks.co.uk

*For the plant spirits,
our beloved teachers Eliot and Alison,
and all of our colleagues, clients and students
with love and gratitude*

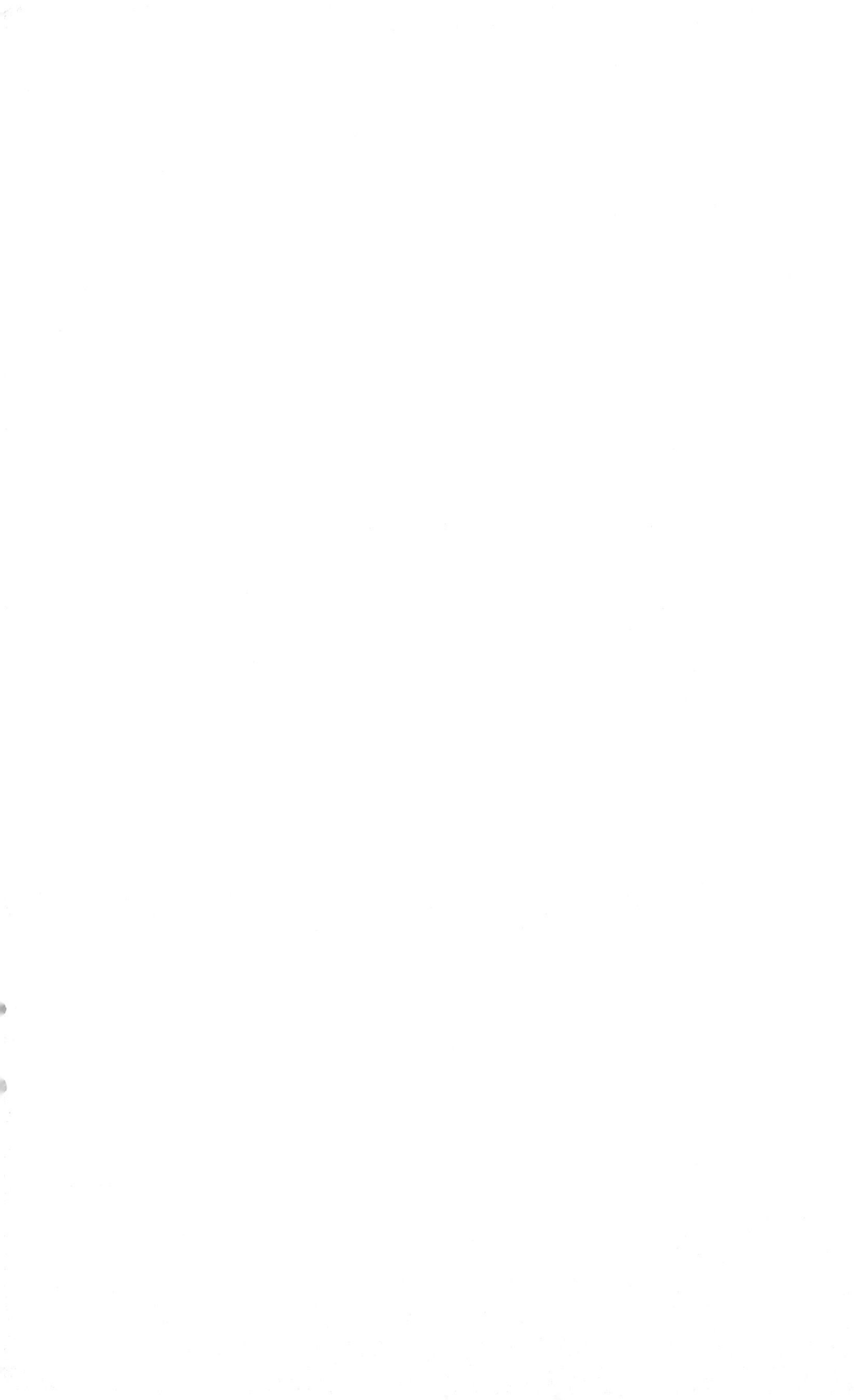

CONTENTS

ACKNOWLEDGEMENTS ix

FOREWORD
By Eliot Cowan xi

INTRODUCTION xv

CHAPTER ONE
A medicine for our time 1

CHAPTER TWO
Plant spirit medicine in practice 21

CHAPTER THREE
Receiving the medicine 41

CHAPTER FOUR
The journey of the seasons 61

CHAPTER FIVE
Meeting the plant spirits—the shamanic dream journey 81

CHAPTER SIX
The healer's journey 105

CHAPTER SEVEN
Called by the plants 125

CHAPTER EIGHT
Journey for the planet 143

CHAPTER NINE
The onward journey—how the plants direct us 161

APPENDIX A—PLANT SPIRIT MEDICINE TODAY 181

APPENDIX B—ACORN MAGIC 189

CONTRIBUTORS 191

ILLUSTRATORS 200

RESOURCES 202

ACKNOWLEDGEMENTS

We would like to thank all those who have made this book possible: first and foremost the plants themselves; all those who generously gave us the stories which make up the heart of this book (they are listed in detail at the back); our teachers of plant spirit medicine, Eliot Cowan and Alison Gayak, and those at the Blue Deer Centre who are working to support the medicine. Special thanks to the lovely Jo Roberts of Chester who took the photograph of the hawthorn flowers and Sofy Descortes of Mexico who took the pic of the beech roots used on the front cover; Oliver, Cecily, Mel, and their design team at Aeon who have published it and made it beautiful. Our gratitude goes out for our people who love the plant spirits as we do, our fellow healers and travellers on the journey and those who let themselves be touched by nature to help bring deep and lasting balance into the future of our world.

FOREWORD

By Eliot Cowan

From the perspective that we hold in plant spirit medicine, which is similar to the perspective that is held in many of what can be called traditional medicines, the state of the world and the state of the people in it is manifesting a lot of problems due to what can be called poor relationship.

Poor relationship to oneself, poor relationship to others, and poor relationship to the world itself. The way people, certainly in the dominant culture, relate to life, and to the world, is very out of balance. People see the world through the eyes of the fears of the mind. The mind sees the world, other people, and even oneself, as presenting endless possibilities for loss and damage and hurt. Somehow we feel that we need to protect ourselves from all that, under the heading of trying to control things. The illusion that you can control things is driven by trying to protect a personal agenda. And that has produced endless amounts of needless destruction, illness, and suffering of various kinds. Because that view doesn't take anything else into account. It doesn't see the world as something that is related to us, that we're part of, and that we can and should have a good relationship to. Not only for our own benefit but for the benefit of others, both humans and the world itself.

We've created a way of life, under the heading of trying to keep ourselves safe, that offers much less safety. Because we are, from the point of view of what can be called ecology, destroying the world and all the relationships and systems of the world which are designed to support us.

Plant spirit medicine in many cases can and does reduce symptoms and so forth. But where does that come from? It comes from a place of people actually having a different experience of their relationship to themselves, their relationship to other humans, and their relationship to the world itself. It starts to bring those things back into balance, which means that it has a very important place in the world and is of great help. Is it the whole enchilada? No, but it's a very important part of it, because it does help to restore something at this deep level that needs to be restored, in a way that just alleviation (temporary, usually) of symptoms doesn't. What's needed is to really solve the problem.

And it does that in a way that's not a theory or a dogma or something that has to be believed. People experience it, they live it. A lot of times they don't know what it is all about, but they live it, they feel it, and that helps to bring that person into better relationship. And guess what, not only does that benefit that individual, but it also benefits all the people whom that individual touches and has relationships with, because they're experiencing something quite different and it produces what could be called a kind of beneficial infection.

There is often an immense benefit for a person's whole family or working companions. People may simply start making better choices and decisions in their lives which affect them and those around them for the better. So I say that besides the beneficial effect on the person we are treating, there's also a beneficial effect on those around that person; and this has a way of spreading, and starting to move things in the direction they have to move to solve these crucial, urgent, dangerous imbalances in the way that we are living that are creating a lot of suffering and a lot of unnecessary destruction.

Here I'm going to relate to another medicine, homeopathy. Without going into a lot of detail, what homeopathy demonstrates is that by a very small intervention, so small that by the standards of Western science it doesn't even exist, a tiny introduction of the appropriate remedy can have effects on the whole system. A good homeopath can give a person a tiny dose and it can change not only his or her state of health but whole life. So in that way I'll say that plant spirit medicine, even though it's small, can and does have a big effect, helping people to move back into a form of living that is much more deeply satisfying and also sustainable, which the current way of life is not.

A good, well told story about plant spirit medicine is medicine itself. Stories touch us in a way that information simply doesn't do. When we hear or read a good story, something in us opens. And something comes through the opening and touches our heart. That's why I say that a plant spirit medicine story gives you a good dose of the medicine.

This is a book of true stories. It's designed to give you many experiences, many healings. Read through it and ask yourself, "What did I learn?" If you expected to learn techniques, you might say, "Well, I didn't learn very much." But I say you will have learned a lot because you will have been touched by a mysterious medicine.

Stories have an enormous effect. That's why in many cultures, the transmission of tradition is done through stories. If you visit indigenous people like those in the Huichol highlands and you think, "I'm going to learn about their medicine," and you expect people to give you a lecture, you won't find it. The way they teach and have always done is the way it has always been done by human beings—through stories.

Information just doesn't touch us the same way. Information speaks to our mind, which is always going to doubt and try to defend itself in the face of something as mysterious as plant spirit medicine. But there is a chasm between experiencing something and thinking about it. So read these stories. Get the experience. Let your heart rejoice in the good medicine here.

INTRODUCTION

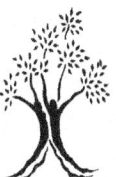

We are in the midst of a quiet revolution, quiet because the plants don't speak out loud. Yet the necessity to listen to them is more urgent than it's ever been, now that we are generally agreed to be on the brink of complete environmental destruction, with human activity as culpable and degraded as at any time in history. Simultaneously there are strong voices telling us we've never had it so good as technology continues to rampage through our lives bringing apparent help whilst it ravages our social relationships and inexorably blocks our essential connection with the natural world.

Although plant spirit medicine, PSM, the subject of this book could simply be seen as yet another natural healing modality, this in no way sufficiently describes its depth, aliveness, and potential impact for us human beings when we engage with it. The astonishing benevolence of the plant spirits is something many of us have become completely oblivious to, just as we are totally unaware of how out of balance we have become as products of an increasingly disconnected society. Although plants continue to give, in unceasing rounds of generosity via food, shelter, and medicine, their gifts have become mere commodities we use up with very little awareness or care of their origins.

As human beings we are busy enough denying our own spiritual natures, so to assert that a plant might even possess a spirit challenges many of us beyond the comfort zone of our current mindset. As organisms with complex physical needs and vulnerabilities we can try to make these the whole picture of being human. We also have another complex and vulnerable aspect, that of the mind, defined in this instance as the mental level of our cognitive functions. It is very specific to humans, having a mind. Other beings don't seem to have much use for one but as humans we need our minds to navigate the world, think, and communicate. Much is known about the complexities of the body and mind these days, it being now generally accepted that the two interrelate and exert a major influence on each other and our overall health. There is, however, a vital ingredient missing in this human recipe, that which gives flavour to the whole being, the indefinable essence that can never be adequately spoken of that is far beyond the reach of the mind. It is felt at key moments when we are fundamentally touched by a clear and heart opening moment: the gaze of a loved one, a stunning sunset, a piece of exquisite music, an awe inspiring landscape, the incredible loveliness of a flower, a peaceful dying breath. Life is spiced with these windows onto what we are calling spirit. Spirit affects the mind as the mind affects the body. Without the health, balance, and radiance of the spirit everything ends up feeling insignificant by comparison, regardless of wealth, success, and relatively good physical health.

We live in times that offer a lot of help and knowledge to heal the body. Unless we are too poor or disadvantaged we have access to medicine that can help our physical bodies. There is also a fair amount of nourishment for our minds: rich culture, wonderful books, theatre and films, fascinating knowledge, and many effective therapies to help heal the mind/psyche. But it is not so easy in our modern world for the life of the spirit to find nourishment and healing. Our societies do a very poor job providing for the health of the spirit. Living without a healthy relationship to spirit separates us from a deep sense of joy, purpose, and fulfilment, so much so that many of us have forgotten these possible qualities in our lives. Such spiritual imbalance needs healing. Plant spirit medicine offers this. We were fortunate enough to learn from a great and inspiring teacher, Eliot Cowan. It was he who coined the term "plant spirit medicine" to describe the medicine he rediscovered, a household shamanic approach to working with the plant spirits in an entirely safe way that didn't involve the same dangers that a deep traditional shamanic path contains. Eliot explains how he came to call the medicine plant spirit medicine;

> Well, by design it's kind of a double entendre. Let me say this first of all: it's a form of doing healing work with plants, but not plants as objects or chemical factories—but as spirit beings, alive and feeling and wise and connected to the world around them, and to ourselves. So it's a way of relating to plants as sources of spiritual healing. We like to say that it is the spirit of the plant that has the unique capacity to touch and heal the spirit of a human being. So it's "plant spirit medicine"—meaning it comes from the spirit of the plant—and it's also "plant spirit medicine," meaning medicine for the spirit of the people who are receivers of their work. (From an interview: www.soundstrue.com/podcast/transcripts/eliot-cowan.php?camefromhome=camefromhome)

If a living butterfly astonishes us by alighting on our hand and we momentarily experience its beauty, we could say that our heart is touched in some way. If we catch the butterfly and pin it inside a display cabinet with its Latin name printed alongside, then our minds think we know something. This knowledge has already removed us from the direct experience of the living butterfly, how we felt in response to being in relationship with it. The mind labels every experience and thereby separates us from true connection with real life.

If ever help was needed to shift us unbalanced humans from our destructive patterns of separation back to a way of living in real relationship with the earth that sustains us, now is the time. This book is our attempt to share the awesome and astonishing depth of plant spirit medicine without pinning it down into a dry, dead thing. We weave together the voices and stories of many people whose lives have been touched by plants in general and plant spirit medicine in particular. These include contributions from some of the many wonderful herbalists using plant-based medicine in a way that goes beyond the physical, biochemical model, and the bulk of the book, the majority of the voices herein, come from those who have been touched by PSM, as reintroduced by Eliot. An ancient medicine which the land knows, which is gently seeding across the world.

The stories are arranged in chapters which take the reader on a journey of discovery of this medicine for our time. It is sometimes said that in the time of greatest need there is the greatest help, and PSM has certainly emerged at a time of great need and challenge and is growing and taking root. The plants themselves, sentient and alive, are calling to many to awaken to a deeper experience of the energy of nature and of our human place in it. This can be felt and understood in direct relationship. The elemental forces that manifest the seasons offer a doorway to move into this perspective. For all the many reasons people may seek out the medicine, there will always be something deep and interesting to learn from an experience of it once we have made the connection. Anyone can learn to communicate directly with plant spirits and befriend them in a way that opens rich dimensions, and over time and with persistence and patience a quiet revolution of perspective can result. Becoming a healer, however, and practising as a healer, is a more committed business that holds as many rewards as it requires dedication, perseverance, and sacrifice. Plant spirit medicine offers the healer the framework of an elegant and rigorous methodology within which to access and effectively channel the energy of the astonishing realm of plant spirits. In the unfolding of our own journeys as healers and receivers of the medicine we witness an unfolding of consciousness in ourselves and our patients which offers something truly hopeful for the journey of the planet.

The plants also have a way of directing us towards the sense of heartfelt purpose a joyful spirit can feel. Acting as stepping stones or bridges, they help us find our paths. Our hope is that with their help our offering does something to illustrate the mysterious beauty and awesome power of this phenomenal medicine.

INTRODUCTION xix

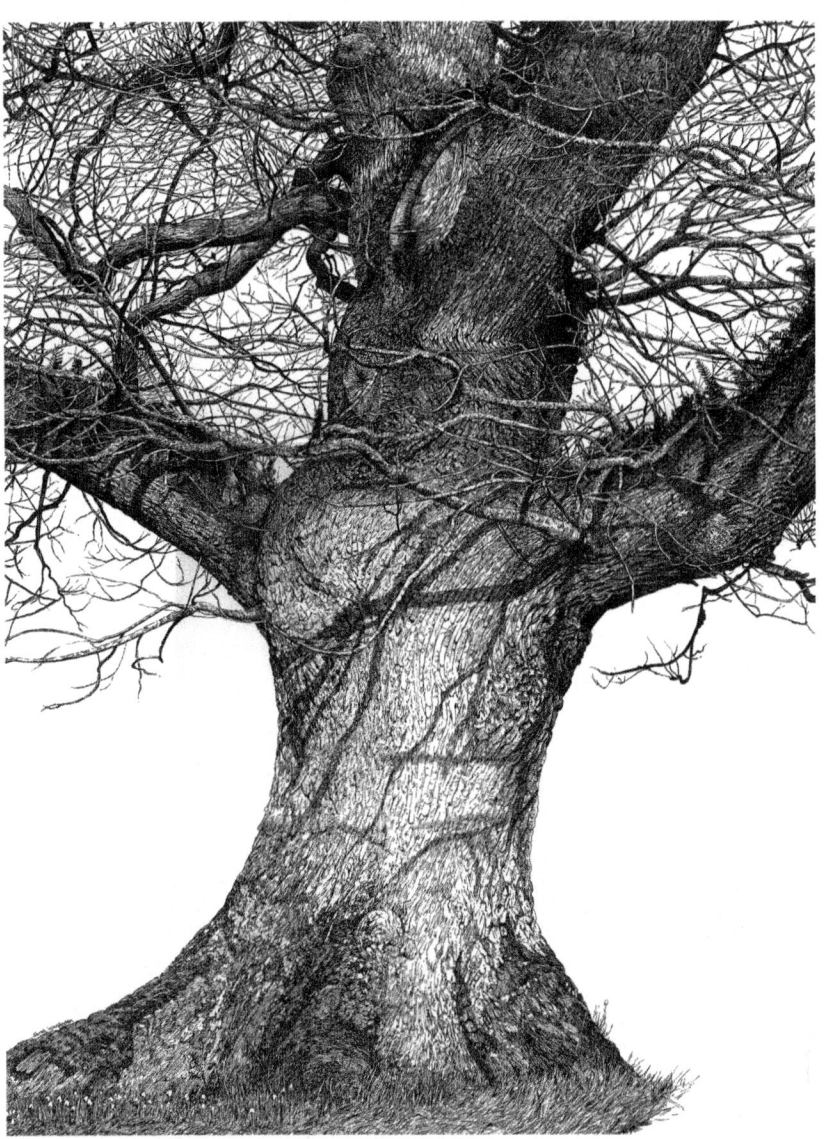

Touch Me Oak by Sarah Woolfenden.

CHAPTER ONE

A medicine for our time

The cars zoom by, the supermarket checkout beeps, we down a quick coffee and do everything to keep business running as usual. How far have we humans travelled into understanding our purpose? How far away from the extraordinarily creative intelligence of the natural world we inhabit? It is not so easy to fully notice the beauty of a so-called weed, bound as we are by crushing time constraints and centuries of conditioning. So what might a small apparently insignificant plant be doing here besides waiting to sting us or irritate an otherwise perfect border or flower bed?

Accidental decoration, oxygen supplier, concrete cracker, future furniture, garden ornament, parks benefactor, beauty supplier, foodstuff, weave potential, herbal wonder: our plant friends are inextricably linked with our lives and our survival, no matter in how many plastic wrappers we try to disguise the fact and deny our dependency. Our minds are used to thinking of plants as commodities for our use along with the earth they and we grow from, the water they and we drink, and the air they and we breathe. Yet since ever there was a need our plant allies have been there to supply it. It is the great good fortune of the authors of this book to be part of an awakening to their great generosity and the deeper gifts they offer.

This awakening is happening alongside the unprecedented environmental destruction of all time, when dozens of species are going extinct every day as a result of human actions—a rate of something like 10,000 times more than happens naturally. Ingrained in us by centuries of conditioning is an all-pervasive superiority complex which insists that humans hold all the answers. It's a big stretch for us to consider that the natural world itself might hold a wisdom and knowing far beyond our own. Our cultural expectations may not enjoy the reminder that we are related to lowly weeds and common or garden plant life, although an amusing fact is that we are said to share up to 60 to 70 per cent of our genes with the oak tree. Our cells and plant cells are extremely similar to look at.

The stuff of our blood, haemoglobin, which enables us to transport the oxygen needed for all our cellular function is almost identical in structure to the chlorophyll which is similarly central to plant physiology—the difference being that haemoglobin is centred upon iron while chlorophyll contains magnesium. How fine it is to have daffodils as our cousins!

And equally wonderful is that modern DNA research has confirmed the long-held knowledge of indigenous peoples: that all life on earth is related. Thomas King, First Nations writer, describing the meaning of the Native saying "for all my relations", puts it beautifully:

> "All my relations" is at first a reminder of who we are and of our relationship with both our family and our relatives. It also reminds us of the extended relationship we share with all human beings. But the relationships that Native people see go further, to the animals, to the birds, to the fish, to the plants, to all the animate and inanimate forms that can be seen or imagined. More than that, "all my relations" is an encouragement for us to accept the responsibilities we have within this universal family by living our lives in a harmonious and moral manner (a common admonishment is to say of someone that they act as if they have no relations). (Thomas King, *All My Relations: An Anthology of Contemporary Canadian Native Fiction*, 1990)

Despite the many nutritional and even herbal uses we modern humans have for plants, we have tended to disinherit them from our human families, convincing ourselves of their inanimate nature and forgetting how to listen to their wisdom. Listening in itself is a poorly practised

A MEDICINE FOR OUR TIME 3

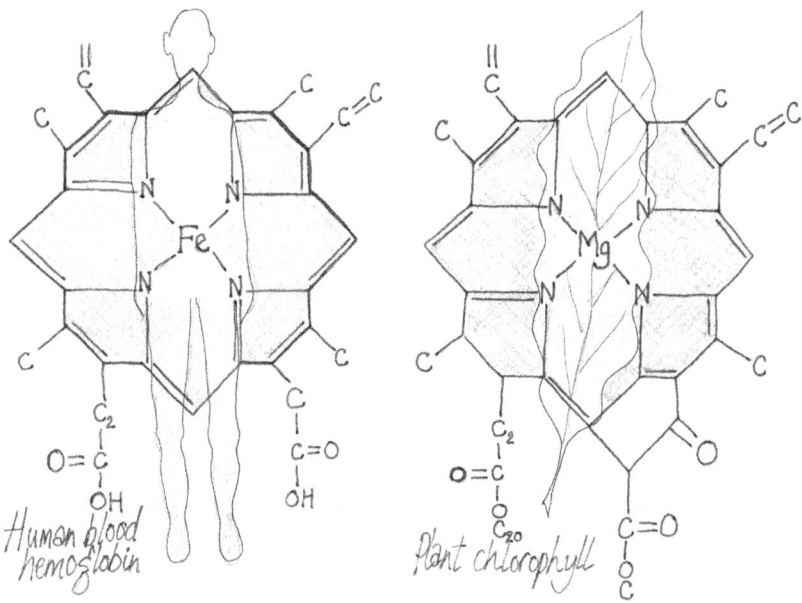

Haemoglobin/Chlorophyll by Lucy Wells.

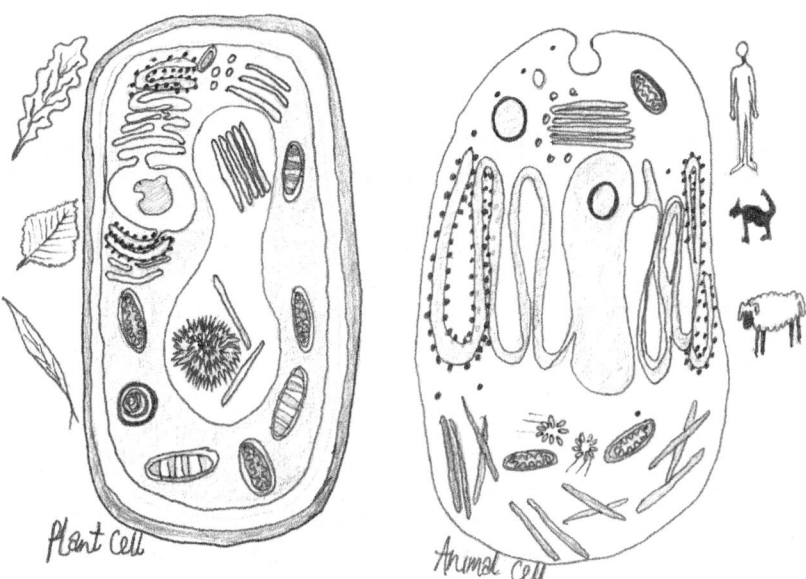

Plant/animal cell by Lucy Wells.

art in the human domain as we are often busy competing to be heard, never mind taking the space to listen to voices in nature. If we ever do stop to think about it, the idea that plants might possess wisdom is still by and large considered the domain of the naive, insane, or misguided. Those who commune deeply with nature may still bear the stigma of suspicion even as most of us seek out beautiful countryside to relax and enjoy ourselves in. High pressured lifestyles are often rewarded with a leafy environment yet how often have the plants themselves been acknowledged and thanked? It has become very well known to "use" plant medicines as healing agents, and gardeners and growers often love their plants, yet there is still a tendency for the plants themselves to be objectified in another form of our insatiable consumerism.

Using a plant-based medicine rather than a drug-based one in an attempt to remove symptoms that arise from the imbalances within our society misses the point. We can't fix things out of the same place that has caused the problem.

Our teacher Eliot Cowan developed *plant spirit medicine* as a natural progression from his practice of five elements acupuncture, his herbal knowledge, and his calling to earth medicine or shamanism. Five elements acupuncture is a healing modality with its roots in ancient China. It is a very distinct and complete medicinal paradigm which sees the cause of disease as being an energetic or spiritual imbalance. The imbalance can be read by signals in the form of colours that are seen in a person's complexion, particularities of body odour, and sound of voice, and something about the emotional flavour—or its lack—with which a person goes through life. Eliot feels that because of his grounding in this elegant and rigorous system of medicine, he was ideally suited to hear the call of the plants. Did the plants call him to plant spirit medicine?

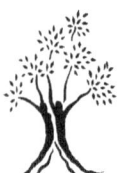

Well, plants often have a feminine way of directing me. Like a wise wife, they make their guidance seem like my own choice. Until I moved to Vermont in my early 20's I had no interest in plants. Suddenly I found them fascinating.

At the time I thought the fascination came from inside me, but looking back, it seems the plants made themselves fascinating as a way of getting me to pay attention to them. They had a lot to show me. Plants on my farm healed my "terminally ill" goat, and this put me in pursuit of natural healing. The pursuit led me to become an acupuncturist. Later I discovered acupuncture had given me a language with which to converse with plants. Those conversations led me to rediscover and bring forth a long-forgotten medicine, which I called Plant Spirit Medicine. Later, an invitation from a sacred plant called the "Wind Tree" showed me I had been called to the healing tradition of the Huichol Indians of Mexico.

Plant spirit medicine involves building relationships with, rather than "using" local plants. It addresses the spiritual and emotional roots of disease. More than simply a healing modality for us struggling humans, it is a path to rediscover our connection with the divine natural world and how to live in it.

When something is described as divine, sacred, or holy we are immediately led into a need for definition and to take a look at our feelings about forces beyond the human. This can be problematic for those who favour a mechanistic world view or who have suffered psychological indoctrination of a particular religious perspective. It seems unavoidable, it really isn't possible for us to approach the subject objectively given our history of bloodshed and hypocritical power abuse in the religious and spiritual domains. The existence or not of gods or divine forces appears to be so highly contentious that it continues to be the cause of ongoing war and bloodshed.

Considering the perfection created in each leaf, snowflake, and insect and animal species, the mystery of our emergence into the world makes a compelling case for a creative force beyond our capacity to name whatever we choose to name it. Moreover, most of us have had at least some experiences in life which are above the ordinary—which touch us in some mysterious way and seem to involve a capacity that is beyond the understanding of materialism.

Whether we are conscious of it or not we are culturally conditioned away from an indigenous perspective that implicitly understands its place in the reciprocal scheme of things. Ours is a world of strong forces that have removed us from connection with the divine elements of nature, leaving us bereft of an easy sense of belonging, purpose, or direction. In truth, we are so very lost that we don't even know there was anything to lose. Plant spirit medicine is a powerful and gentle antidote to this. Through relationship with the plants, the healer matchmakes between patients and their plant allies which are able to offer us what we really need. Their profound and mysterious capacities promote movement towards greater balance and harmony on all levels.

There are various ways of describing the innate energy of a plant—plant spirits, plant awareness, plant consciousness, and so on. All refer to the same thing—that same life-force or soul that we understand as inseparable from the body of the plant, just as our own spirits are inseparable from our bodies while life is within us. But what actually is *plant spirit medicine*? It can be understood as a medicine, a help or healing, from the plant spirits and to our spirits. But what do these words invoke in us? In the mixed soup that is our modern culture, there is much diverse interpretation, assumption, and cultural difference in experience that affects how we hear words. When we are in a group introducing people to plant spirit medicine, we explore what people understand by these words. It's not a test, and is entirely subjective, but as a way of starting from scratch so we can get on the same page it's interesting to hear how we make associations and thereby also assumptions.

The word "plant" can conjure anything between green growing thing and dig-into-the-ground, and lots beside and beyond: friend, tree, help, food, weed, root, ally, messenger, beauty, herb, flower, everywhere, compost, leaf, growing child of nature, medicine, poison, compost, jungle, rainforest, chlorophyll, photosynthesis, oxygen, necessary. Such a wide range of interpretation from one simple word.

The word "spirit" can evoke ghosts, the unseen force, the ether, energy and soul, that which underlies everything; as well as whisky or any other good stiff drink, invisible, chi, dynamism, that which cannot be named, and willpower. It feels important that we find some level ground from which to launch our inquiry and besides, it's a great game to play with words and clarify communication so we can learn from each other what we actually understand.

The word "medicine" elicits an equally wide response from yuck to healing, doctor to pill, power to disease, and causes us to mentally range through hospital, drug, sick, well, health, elixir, poison, answer, placebo, alternative, natural, pharmaceutical, and making things better. This word, medicine, has a much deeper meaning in many indigenous cultures than it does in our own. For many indigenous peoples of the Americas, including Canada, who comprise many distinct tribes, the word has a much broader and richer meaning than simply something used to treat disease or enhance wellness. Medicine refers to the energy of a person, place, object, natural force, or event—the "energy" can mean its presence, its power, its spirit—that which is intrinsically there within a person, animal, plant, rock, place, or other thing. This can be seen also as its mystic potency or innate qualities that go well beyond its physical or external appearance. *It is this indigenous idea of medicine that is meant by our use of the word "medicine" as we talk about the plants.*

This is not an easy concept to put across in words on a page. We will not pin down the butterfly. Words point towards knowing, but they can't lead us to wisdom. It takes experience to do this. The indigenous view is more experiential, more of the body and senses. It actually is impossible to experience it while reading a book—yet we hope here to give you a taste of its trail, and more than that, a yearning to take things further and build your own relationships with the plants. However much you have already been touched by nature, our prayer is to be part of opening that door still further. So now, before proceeding further, put the book down and find a living plant.

Our world, and our plants, are in increasing danger from the relentless consumerism that characterises much of our human endeavour. Unprecedented numbers of humans are living on the earth today, and perhaps the majority of these live in ways far removed from nature. The lost words of our time are a striking illustration of how far and fast we in the UK are moving in this direction. The most up-to-date English children's dictionary has had to drop more and more

> If you are able to, go outside and find a plant which is growing of its own volition (rather than one planted although trees are a happy exception, being old enough to have outgrown the human intervention). If you can't get outside, sit with a house plant. Allow yourself the moments to observe your leafy cousin and be together as if you'd made a date. Notice your feelings, notice your breathing, notice the machinations of your mind (which might hate this exercise!), and notice the plant; its structure, form, colours, shape, way of relating to its environment, and so on. After some minutes, see if anything has changed—how do you feel now in your body? How do you feel emotionally?

vocabulary as the new words of our technology-rich culture multiply. We lost almond, blackberry, and crocus, replaced by analogue, block graph and celebrity in the Oxford Junior Dictionary in 2007. Catkin, chestnut, and acorn also got axed, giving way to cut and paste, chat room, and attachment. This is expressed with exquisite art and poetry in Robert Macfarlane's beautiful children's book, *The Lost Words* (2017).

At the same time, many are aware of how important it is for us to regain, and retain, our sense of connection with nature. Japanese studies of the practice of shinrin-yoku, forest bathing, or spending time in natural green spaces, show that this pastime reduces the stress hormone cortisol, calms the brain, helps the cardiovascular system, and boosts immunity. The Japanese are leading in this type of research—a 2008 study published in the *Journal of the Japanese Society for Horticultural Science* even showed that high school classrooms filled with potted plants for a four-month trial period significantly reduced visits to the infirmary compared with age-matched students attending classes without the visible plants! Variations on this study have been repeated in other countries with similar results, including showing improved grades for maths and science! And closer to home, forest schooling is becoming increasingly popular as educators realise the power of the natural world to facilitate healthy learning.

According to Dr Miles Richardson, head of psychology at the University of Derby, there is research evidence that proves exposure to nature can reduce hypertension, reduce respiratory and cardiovascular illnesses, improve vitality and mood, improve depression and anxiety, restore attention capacity, and relieve mental fatigue. He conducted a study looking at 18,500 people who took on "doing something wild" every day for 30 days. Feeling a part of nature has been shown to significantly correlate with life satisfaction, vitality, meaningfulness, happiness, and mindfulness, and lower cognitive anxiety. Fully 30 per cent more people reported their health as being "excellent" after the period of the study—and many of them loved it so much they continued on afterwards. "These correlations are of a similar magnitude to those found between wellbeing and other variables, such as marriage and education, whose relationships with wellbeing are well established" (Richardson, Cormack, McRobert, & Underhill, 2016). He adds that recent analysis found people with a stronger connection to nature experienced more life satisfaction, positive affect, and vitality at levels associated with established predictors of satisfaction, such as personal income. "There is a need to normalise everyday nature as part of a healthy lifestyle."

Lucy McRobert of the Wildlife Trust who was a partner in the research says, "Nature isn't a miracle cure for diseases, but by interacting with it, spending time in it, experiencing it and appreciating it we can reap the benefits of feeling happier and healthier as a result." All who love plants and the outdoors know this through their own experience; however, those of us who work with plants as healers know they have infinitely more to offer than is yet fully realised—a lifetime working with them only ever reveals more that is still unknown. While we in the modern world are far removed from the nature that sustains all life, working with plant spirits or allies has been part of every indigenous culture's healing toolkit. Just as the bodies of plants have been used for healing our bodies since human and animal time began, so there has always been an understanding of the spiritual assistance that plant spirits offer.

Indigenous peoples are those who still live (or try to live, given the constraints of the era) in their original homeland, with at least some flavour of the ways, customs, language, and spiritual traditions that remain available to them. These are as varied as there are peoples but all involve a deep understanding and connection with and of the land, which is respected as sacred. The earth of place is the flesh and bones of the people and ancestors; language is brought forth from the ground to the tongue via the heart; an understanding of being human involves the responsibility of stewardship and reciprocation with place rather than domination and usage.

In "Rediscovering What Has Always Been There" Glenn H. Walker (www.indigenouspeople.net) sums up the indigenous perspective:

> When will we ever begin to understand the meaning of the soil underneath our feet? From a tiny grain of sand to the largest mountain, everything is sacred. Our living saints are the evergreen trees. We have no buildings or steeples. The landscape and lakes are our churches and cathedrals. These are our sacred buildings. Yesterday and tomorrow exist forever upon our mother, the earth.

Eliot Cowan (*Plant Spirit Medicine*, 2014) writes.

> Once we were all indigenous—but centuries (or even millennia) of conquest and domination have seriously fragmented or completely obliterated most original cultures so we no longer understand an indigenous perspective even if we are living in the country we were born in, where all our ancestors were born. We have become soul mutts with our genealogy and place of birth no longer being reliable guides to what our soul is made up of.

Sadly for the majority of the world's population, what indigenous actually means has been lost in a series of land thefts, genocides, market force imperatives, and an ignorant sense of superiority. What we have naively labelled progress has caused widespread devastation and in fact has led us in the so-called first world to the brink of destruction where technology threatens to make being human redundant. Some might say it serves us right. There are few remaining indigenous peoples who have managed to keep their traditions intact. Despite having to defend their rights to exist on their land as global imperialism lusts for more, they still hold a treasure store in their knowing of their place in the grand scheme of things, and work with the plants and animals, waters, earth, mountains, and sky as a matter of spiritual necessity. For such an extreme and enormous imbalance that we see played out daily in so many ways on our newsfeeds, a serious medicine is needed. Plant spirit medicine as a direct link to the natural world offers not only the immeasurable healing power of plants but also a way of really hearing what a person's spirit is crying out for.

As in original indigenous practice, our important plant allies in plant spirit medicine are those seemingly humble plants we live among, the ones that pop up in the cracks in the pavement or populate the hedgerow. Exotic plants from afar, which have enormous relevance for their own people, may seem to offer a quick and powerful fix out of our own messes, but can often bring us unwanted trouble. The trend in their use seems to be part of a misguided colonial spiritual consumerism. The plants we need spring up outside our back doors or in the tarmac of our cities. These know us as neighbours of the same earth, and want us to step up and take responsibility, call upon their help, and recognise and respect their gifts. As they have told more than one of the pioneer healers of our time, they have been waiting—it is time for their call to be heard by many. It is indeed a case of rediscovering what has always been there.

The plants are contacting us all the time, reminding us of our true place, that of being in relationship with all of the natural world. This can happen in so many ways: from a simple need to walk in the woods to restore mental equilibrium, to a deeply connected use of their energy to unravel complex problems on all levels of our bodies, minds, and spirits. I (Lucy) didn't realise the relationships I was building as I would do my daily tai chi practice under a tree in the park or the garden. It didn't really occur to me that as I was endeavouring to help my internal life force relax and flow the trees were aware of my being. As I became more horrified by the impact of rampant consumerism and the damage we were perpetrating on our living world a number of significant incidents happened in my life that led to an awareness that the troubles we might experience in our own lives were being mirrored on a vast and destructive scale in the world we are a part of. And the trees and other plants let me know they were intelligent and cognisant of this and, astoundingly, given modern humanity's greed, were more than willing to help. What a time to have such friends.

While training as a medical herbalist in the 1980s in a Western school which relied almost exclusively on the scientific paradigm and a knowledge of the active chemicals in plants to explain their healing actions, I (Pip) came across a way of relating to plants as fellow beings with their own unique personalities and ways to heal that went deeper than their pharmacology. I had the good fortune to work for a while with Elisabeth Brooke, a herbalist with a deep interest in the more magical aspects of herbalism (see her *A Woman's Book of Herbs*, 1992). Elisabeth is an astrologer and tarot expert and uses this understanding in her work. She taught a type of mindfulness meditation or Goethean method of paying close attention to the taste, smell, and feel of a dried plant; tasting the tea and noticing all effects of this—where you felt it in your body, emotions that came up, colours, chakras, and so on, followed by a guided meditation or visualisation. It was a very useful approach, to begin to feel that the plants were friends and allies in the healing process, more than just a bottle of jollop that interacted chemically with the human body. It certainly sharpened my "feel" for which plants to choose for which patients—and this was nice. However, although I am grateful for the introduction to connecting with plants that working with Elisabeth gave me, I never had a feeling for an astrological paradigm. I couldn't really connect it with the other herbal knowledge I had acquired.

The lack of a distinct diagnostic framework in which to use this extra dimension of understanding meant that for many years I practised with a sometimes frustrating feeling that I wasn't quite reaching people where they most needed to be reached. This rumbled away through years, as I learned more about the necessity for emotional healing, and began a rich exploration of earth medicine or shamanic healing which I was very attracted to having always been more of an Indian than a cowboy.

After some years of following these threads, things started to get interesting and I was led to study plant spirit medicine by a series of mysteriously magical events. Now after fourteen years of immersion in the medicine, it has become the mainstay of what I do, and my experience of it being a very important offering for the perilously unbalanced times we are living in continues to deepen and grow. In it I have found the deep healing that I always sensed was needed—for myself, for my patients, and for the troubled world.

There has been a great upward surge of interest in natural medicine in recent decades, with many high-level training courses available in plant-based medicinal systems including herbalism of many sorts, naturopathy, and homeopathy (which doesn't only but primarily uses plant energies to potentiate remedies). In the field of herbal medicine there is a strong trend to follow the biochemical materialistic model that is dominant in our culture, with herbs seen as complex drugs, their usefulness dependent on their chemical constituents. Of course oftentimes we need physical support for the body's processes, and today's leading herbalists have found many ways to work beyond a one-dimensional approach. As herbalists know, there is an incredibly rich and complex dimension to the chemistry of a single herb. Plants are the alchemists of the natural world. They take in ingredients from the soil, breaking them into atoms and molecules and building their own astonishing biochemistry in response to the conditions they find themselves growing in. Stephen Harrod Buhner explores this in his many fine books on plant medicine. In *The Lost Language of Plants* (2002) he gives a list of 129 known active ingredients found in a single yarrow plant and eloquently describes not only plant chemistry but the way this diversity interacts with local environments to keep health and balance amongst all species and for the land itself:

> As long as the plants are promiscuously producing compounds that regularly fall in a resource cascade to the ground, the battery remains full, the soil rich and bountiful. Through tightly coupled

feedback processes information on the chemistry reserves stored in humic acid feeds back into the aboveground plant communities, indicating what plants should grow in what combination in what ecosystem and what kinds of chemistries they should produce to keep the soil healthy.

Many herbalists today understand the limitations of the purely biochemical perspective and experience plants in a broader way, practising herbal medicine from a deeper perspective. Matthew Wood sums it up in his *The Book of Herbal Wisdom* (1997): "To feel the living spirit and intelligence of nature is the true foundation for developing a knowledge of herbal medicine."

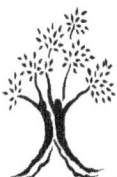

My approach to healing encompasses an understanding about life. I believe that all of nature is alive—every single individual plant has its own life force. And that has an ability to communicate and respond to other life forces. As humans, we are part of nature. So when I work with people, both patients and students, the beginning premise is that all of life can intercommunicate, interconnect, and interact together. My formal clinical training as a medical herbalist was devoid of this. We were looking at very physical or material ideas, and it left me a bit bereft. I was quite unhealthy, especially emotionally and mentally, during my training. Now as I leave my house and walk up my garden path and past the aromatics, I never pass them without touching them and saying "Good morning". And when I walk down the road in my village I greet each and every one of the trees and plants by name, and it gives me a sense of wholeness and a sense of rooted connectedness to my place. And I just wish this for each and every one of the people that come to me for healing, that they can have this sense of rooted connection to the place they are living in. **Karen Lawton, sensory herbalist and hopeful activist, UK**

At university (studying herbal medicine) I met Karen; we were both into play and fun and exploring and experimenting, and we would go out together, collect and harvest herbs, talk to the plants, talk to each other, get our feeling about what they might be useful for and go afterwards and do research. It was from those direct experiences with the plants that I think becoming a healer really happened. You can learn all of the anatomy and physiology and biochemistry and botany in the world, but if you don't know the plants, if you haven't connected with them in a spiritual, more direct hands-on way, something of the magic is lost. For me the essence of "healer" is to find solace in nature, connect with the plants themselves, and bring the messages of the plants to people. For us it was very much about being led by the plants themselves. **Fiona Heckels, sensory herbalist and hopeful activist, UK**

Of all the terms referring to plant spirits, plant people, plant beings, mostly I use the term *plant consciousness*. The plant is and always has been all that, so to separate off an aspect as being different or distinct fails to express the fundamental intrinsic quality of the plants, that they are and always have been conscious and intelligent beings. They have a history far broader and deeper than our own history as humans. The main, most powerful healing I see happening when working with a plant is that people open up to their own web of interconnectedness and the energy that's available to them through that web. In the process they integrate realms of internalised trauma that have cut them off from that web. I think many disease processes stem from a breakdown in that interconnectedness and the illusion of separateness by the creation of lives that are deeply programmed to be separate by the values of our culture. The plants have a way of reminding us that that isn't reality, it's just a human construct. They remind us spiritually, they remind our bodies, they remind us emotionally. It's as if they take us back to a truer state of being that we've separated ourselves from.

The main word guiding my work is "relationship"; to aspects of self, to the land, to our food, and really importantly to the medicine. It's harder and harder for me to give a generic bottle of tonic as I might have done ten years ago. What I know is possible is that individuals can be in relationship with the plant they're working with and through that relationship something shifts within them. The crucial factor in the healing dynamic is not getting the right herb and the quantity, it's the depth and the possibilities within the relationship. And then they work with it a while and in that process there's an unfolding. So it's all about an awareness of the intelligence of living nature, an openness to develop relationships with the plants, and with patients. This goes deeper than the medical story of the person's "presenting complaint". **Nathaniel Hughes, herbalist and founder of the School of Intuitive Herbalism, UK**

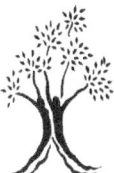

It is possible to practise herbal medicine in a way that respects and recognises the innate intelligence of the plant and the hidden roots beneath the surface of our particular concerns. This type of herbal medicine is a vast improvement on mechanistic medicine. It is echoed in the toolkits of many indigenous healers and their Western heirs and its resurgence now is part of the call to wholeness which the plant people are singing from every forest and meadow, hedgerow and herb garden.

We are living in times when increasing demand for herbal medicines now threatens many wild populations of these plants. Responsible herbalists are aware of this—the problem comes from over-the-counter sales of herbs rather than prescribed medicines from practising herbalists. But still the focus on symptoms and their removal seeps into all aspects of our minds and lives. Almost all of our emotions have become, or are becoming, medicalised. Exuberant two and three year olds are drugged to allow them to settle in classrooms and be biddable in a world that doesn't meet their needs. A person still sad a mere two weeks after the death of a loved one can be officially diagnosed as a candidate for antidepressants. When we are grieving, we might rather take St John's wort for our "low mood" than Prozac or other pharmaceuticals. But as the real "cure" for grief is to simply feel it, to do the work of grieving, letting ourselves feel the truth of the experience of loss, then any attempt to suppress or avoid this quintessentially human feeling is another step on the path to being numb, shut down, and becoming another foot soldier in the army of the zombie apocalypse. Plant spirit medicine healers learn to view and understand emotion in a different way—we learn in our training that as humans we are always feeling something—balance does not mean an absence of feeling, rather we begin to feel more appropriately in response to any given life situation. We recover the innate ability to move from one emotion to another. The judgement of the emotional spectrum is an aspect of our conditioning that is so ingrained we generally don't even notice ourselves and each other's incessant repression and denial.

The plants are calling us to wake up, to really live. They offer their love, their friendship, and their indescribable mysterious assistance again and again in an outpouring of extraordinary generosity. Working in the vast and unfathomable realm of spirit, the plants themselves deliver healing gently and persistently to the source of our imbalance, giving what it is lacking.

All the stories in this book describe in one way or another the effects of encounters with plant spirits. They are in no way exhaustive and do not attempt to prove anything, but if storytelling is the original and best way to learn about life and its challenges then we hope that this may prove true for learning about the potential of the plant spirits as healers for our people at this time. For many people the results can be profound yet very subtle. On rare occasions the results are so dramatic and astounding that they become truly unforgettable.

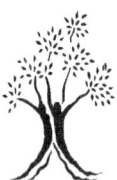

I first went for plant spirit medicine just over seven years ago, having been recommended by a few different people, and I'm so glad I did! Not only did it permanently sort out the physical problem that I presented my healer with but I feel as though that first day was a turning point in my life. Whatever it is (still a bit of a mystery to me!) it really works on all sorts of levels. I now go back for occasional courses of treatment seasonally and that always puts me back on track and gives a bit of perspective. I hope I can keep on benefiting for a long time to come.

Plant spirit medicine saved my life literally. I was very sick when I met my plant spirit medicine healer, and she nurtured me back to a tolerable life. I haven't a clue how it worked but as each week passed I started to feel better and better. I am eternally grateful. Not only did she facilitate my healing but she showed me a way forward to improve my life dramatically. It has been a long haul—but then it took a long haul to get as ill as I was.

A very sincere and thoughtful young woman, "Sameera", came to see me for treatments around twelve months after attending one of my plant spirit medicine talks. I noticed the great trouble she had walking into my office on her crutches. Speaking with her I learned this was the result of a neurological disorder, the main symptoms being involuntary muscle contractions that make controlling her limbs very difficult. Things had become so bad for her that she had mostly been confined to a wheelchair for several months. I observed how grief stricken she was. She carried tremendous grief from the conflict in the Middle East that had affected her extended family. She was also grieving the strained relationships with her immediate family, in particular her father. She was unable to talk for more than a few minutes at a time without breaking into long, deep sobs. The plant that I chose is a tiny little flower that thrives in the sandy, coastal plains of where I live in Western Australia. When I journeyed with this plant, its way to offer its medicine was to have me sob uncontrollably for ten minutes. It seemed like the perfect plant for the occasion! Within a few weeks of treatments Sameera's health improved rapidly and she no longer needed crutches. With continued treatments her sobbing softened and reduced, more joy and laughter arose in her life. Her family relationships were still strained, the situation in the Middle East continued, but she now had an inner strength to deal with the previously overwhelming pain. I still remember taking a phone call from Sameera one day while she was on holiday in central Australia. She rang me with joy in her voice, letting me know that she had blisters on her feet! That day she had walked around the base of Uluru, the spectacular red monolith in the central desert, a distance of nearly 10 km. Her healing continued for many months until I got another phone call after she had taken a long road trip up the coast of Western Australia. As soon as she and her friends left their campsite, and began driving back home, her symptoms began to return. By the time she arrived home she was again unable to walk. I visited her that night, and gave her a treatment, but this time the plants didn't seem to reach her. The subsequent treatments I gave her only brought temporary relief from the symptoms. I learned that she had brought home some beautiful stones from the remote beaches up north, a collection that filled two or three large jars. I knew that one of the ancient laws of the aboriginal ancestors of this land is that no one is allowed to remove stones from the land. I suspected that the ancestors were calling Sameera to return the stones and their message was sent via her worsening symptoms. As helpful as the plants had been, there was very little they could do until Sameera had rectified her relationship with the ancestors and returned the stones. She was very sceptical when she heard my diagnosis. But after several weeks of worsening symptoms she was ready to try. She was unsure whether she had the stamina to undertake this journey as she was barely able to walk at all. The journey would require a long two day drive to the campsite and at least a 2 km walk to the beach where the stones came from. I advised her to trust the ancestors. If they wanted her to return the stones they would help and support her. Several days later Sameera came over for a treatment. She walked into my office and seemed much better. Her quest was successful: the ancestors approved of her work and the plants were again able to support her as before. Every spring this tiny plant bursts into yellow flowers and my heart leaps in awe and gratefulness for its incredible medicine and belonging to this land. **Phil Roberts, PSM healer and SFC fire keeper, Australia**

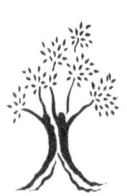

Plant spirit medicine addresses the knowing that something is amiss, even though we might not be able to really put our finger on it. There is an immeasurable benefit in receiving this gift from the divine plant world. Healing from plant spirits is not new. Its re-emergence is part of the needed wisdom and guidance for a proper and sustainable way of living as humans on our beautiful planet. For this reason it is indeed a medicine for our time.

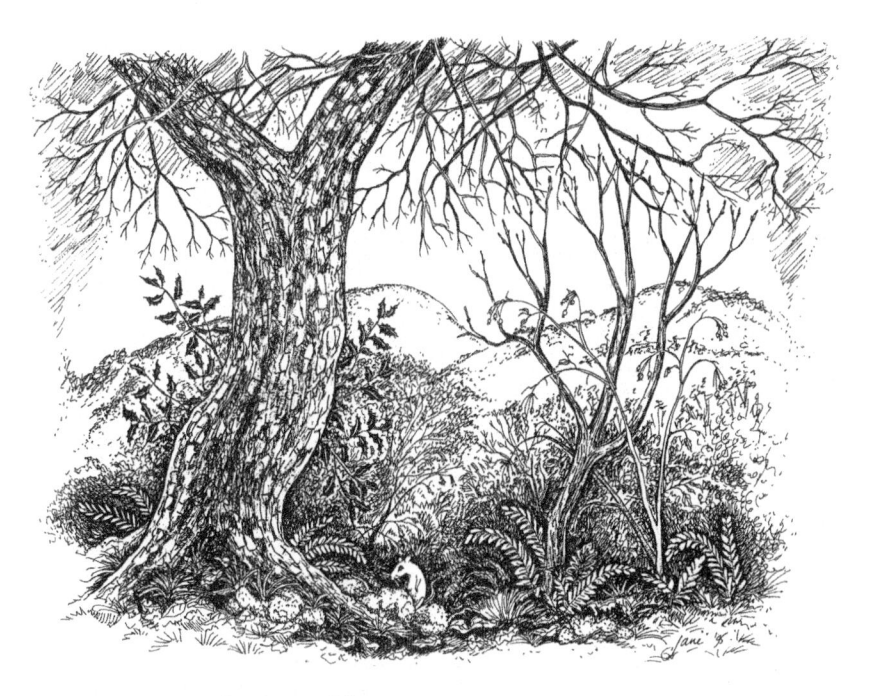

Woodland Scene by Jane Tibbotts.

CHAPTER TWO

Plant spirit medicine in practice

There are so many beautiful approaches to healing generally, and to delivering plant medicine specifically. Herbal, homeopathic, and plant essences are generally given to people to ingest. Doses range from heroically high amounts through to drop doses of herbal tinctures and to the highly diluted potencies of homeopathic remedies, which although no longer containing significant levels of the actual chemical remedy carry a powerful charge of its energetic essence. It is clear that the "spirit" of the plant can be fully at work in the way these medicines operate, just as the physical body of the herb, in whatever amount, acts upon the body. We give full respect to those herbalists who work with plants in this deep way, and to those who call on the spirits of plants as healing agents within other traditions.

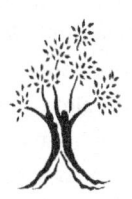

Through my connection with the land and all of the various beings who live here, including the plants and human ancestors, I have cultivated a deep relationship with both the physical and spiritual aspects of the world where I live. All aspects of my practice as an herbalist are guided by this: I only work with a particular plant medicine if the spirit of the plant calls me to work with it; this involves asking permission and making prayer and tobacco offerings when harvesting the herbs, macerating and pressing tinctures, etc. When I'm working with a client the spirits guide me in preparing their formula. We are using their bodies (the tincture) as a physical vehicle through which they are able to provide for the people in body, heart, mind, and spirit. I don't tell the spirits what that is supposed to look like. They know what the people need. **Michael Vertolli, herbalist, Canada**

An infant was brought to me, the family was distraught. He had had a parietal (brain) haemorrhage. They were prepared by the doctors that he was going to be disabled. I placed my hands on the child and felt the yew breathing through the child. A few days later or so they went for another scan, the haemorrhage had completely vanished. It wasn't me of course it was the yew. **Michael Dunning, Yew Shaman, USA**

After working with somebody with severe endometriosis for a while we found that her body was holding an incredible degree of trauma related to very early heart surgery. There was a complete disconnect and almost a hatred or disgust at her own heart. Over many years, and through a lot of work with rose, hawthorn as well, but rose was the big feature of this process, she finally came to a place where she feels like she likes her own heart. That was an immense threshold to move through and I feel sure that it wouldn't have been possible without the plants. There's something to do with an acceptance and a gentleness and love, self-love. It's almost like the plants have been whispering these possibilities over years and years and years, and then at some point there's a critical mass. These presences show that they have some kin to this person's being and something is fundamentally changed. **Nathaniel Hughes, herbalist and founder of the School of Intuitive Herbalism, UK**

The Western allopathic approach is the dominant paradigm understood in our culture as medicine. It is at the same time enormously effective in many circumstances, sometimes depressingly useless and at worst, harmful. This isn't a paranoid assertion. The official statistics reveal that iatrogenic disease—that caused by doctor or hospital treatments—accounts for 9.5 per cent of all deaths, the third leading cause of death in the USA (heart disease and cancer being the first two at around one in three deaths each).

Allopathic medicine has a purely materialistic approach to health and disease, the body seen and investigated as a complex bit of machinery, reduced to parts either working, failing, or wearing out. When something goes wrong it's because there is some kind of malfunction in normal processes. Diagnosed diseases often involve simply a (usually Latin) name of what is going on. For example "tonsilitis" means simply that the lymphoid glands of the throat are inflamed. Underlying causes of disease describe only what is happening in the tissues—the cause could be an infectious agent, a genetic abnormality, degeneration from age, cancer, and so on. Many diseases, seen from a Western allopathic perspective, have an unknown aetiology (cause).

Many of us as patients have been frustrated in the hands of the system which separates all our different body parts—even in the orthopaedic hospital, for example, you see one department for your hips and another for your knees.

Holistic paradigms attempt to see the human being as a whole person living in relationship to all aspects of environment. Indeed there is increasing movement within Western allopathic medicine itself to try to join things up. Some diseases confound categorisation and require collaboration between different departments. For example the connective tissue problem Ehlers Danloss syndrome (EDS) which can affect every system of the body creates huge challenges for the mainstream orthodox system which doesn't yet know how to respond.

Western herbal medicine uses a basis of anatomy, physiology, and pathology alongside understanding of plant chemistry to treat disease, often effectively and certainly without the high cost of drugs and surgery that allopathic medicine extracts. There is a great need for this kind of natural approach to the relief of our human suffering. But this is still symptomatic relief and rarely addresses what is underneath the call of our symptoms. Plant spirit medicine as a healing modality requires a shift of perspective regarding symptoms and the causes of disease. We seek to discover what the spirit is crying for beneath the alarm flag of the symptoms. The diagnostic approach is separate from the story of the disease, because two people with the same illness can be crying out for completely different medicine.

Although it is impossible to really separate body and spirit, the plant spirits don't actually need a physical vehicle to do their work and be powerfully effective—the healer who has built a relationship previously with a plant knows how to call on it to bestow its medicine on a patient. This call is made via our hearts, without any physical vehicle such as a tincture, tea, essence, or pill to carry the healing power of the plant. Remedies cannot be taught one healer to another because each one needs to build his or her own relationship with the plants in order to be able to call on them as medicinal agents. In the practice room we literally put our hands on our patients and make a request for help in line with protocols previously agreed to and empowered by initiation as part of our training.

There are healers everywhere who understand the connection made by direct relationship; the innovation of PSM is to marry the request of the plant spirits to be reintroduced with an extremely thorough diagnostic and feedback system. This is the traditional Chinese five elements approach which was pioneered in the UK by acupuncturist Professor J. R. Worsley.

Over the years since the 1990s when Eliot began to be more public with his work, many offshoots and parallel discoveries have grown in the field. The term *plant spirit medicine* has become for many a general term, just as *herbal medicine* refers to many philosophies and methods. I myself (Pip) had assumed that this was all it was, until I studied plant spirit medicine at its source and experienced it transforming my life and my practice which had been mostly one of herbal medicine for the sixteen years previously. For me, immersing myself in the very complete diagnostic methodology of five elements medicine was revolutionary. I had to get over some prejudices to do this—I had a story in my mind that it was foreign to me, having its roots in China which I never felt a strong affinity for. The case I had built against "Chinese medicine" in my mind occluded my ability to see that although it has its roots in that country, it goes far beyond human ideas of culture. Its insights and wisdom apply wherever nature is found. One tragedy for those of us of European descent is that we have long lost our own ancient traditional ways, including those of our medicine. The path of deep nature connection through the wheel of the year that the five elements paradigm offers is a reliable and time proven doorway. As a particularly exacting system of medicine based on thousands of years of critical observation of how the elemental energies make up all that lives in the world, it requires a refined use of all the senses, an ability to see and hear beyond the story into that same elemental field and an awareness of how the chi (or vital life force) moves through a human being following specific pathways. It describes disease in terms of relative balance and imbalance and seeks to move towards balance and harmony, a place that the plant spirits are perfectly attuned to.

Emotional fluency as an important aspect of the practice of plant spirit medicine is no mean feat for the healer in a society where suppression of feelings is the norm and the way things are set up make it increasingly difficult to relate to nature. In fact the flow of appropriate emotional response is key to moving towards not only a fuller and more enriching life experience on the personal level, but is essential to save our world from human mismanagement. If this seems a far-fetched claim, consider the emotional health of many of our world leaders. We see on the world stage writ large the imbalances we experience in our own hearts. Likewise the more we are aligned with our heart's promptings the greater our contribution for serving the greater healing which is so needed. Alongside the accumulation of the techniques used for diagnosis and delivery of PSM, what healers are invited to learn as part of our training is a dramatic shift in perspective and world-view. It is the experiencing of the living butterfly and refusal to pin it down. This demands humility, and is a challenge to our notion of control and thirst for investigation at the expense of inhabiting the mystery. The mental level of our mind is seriously confronted, attached as it is to nailing everything down.

Consider just how difficult our world finds it to honour wintertime with the quiet it calls for. There is little let-up in routines that might be easy in fuller warmth and light. Stress gets created when dark and cold cause contraction and the wish or need to hibernate is ignored. The natural inclination inwards for restoration, introspection, and stillness is offering us the most precious opportunity yet our current lifestyles often won't allow it. Business always has to be as usual. Many of us have even forgotten that this quiet need exists or are trapped into financial situations that simply don't give time for rest, and we wonder why we might lack energy or fall sick. Plants on the other hand have these cycles at the heart of their being.

The full power of spring energy is more popular with our current world-view. Growth is seen as a positive force particularly in the economic market place where productivity and consumption are actively encouraged to increase. In fact if this increase isn't constant then there is an extra push to keep it going, and thus we see the rampant and overbearing, out of control continual growth that loses sight of what is reasonable, decent, and humane, such as in the cruel treatment in animal husbandry, the desecration of woodland and forests, and the plunder, pillage, and devastation of war for natural resources.

Still in the midst of all of this who amongst us doesn't wish to be loved, to blossom and flower, and be seen in our beauty? Yet how lacking is this deep and vibrant joy that allows us to deeply connect with the vitality of our life's purpose and each other. So many of us are not sure what to do, whether in fact we have anything to offer, in order to understand our meaning. Depression and other mental health issues are epidemic, the full and easy light of summertime absent.

Despite the rise in awareness in healthy eating and countless celebrity chefs, it is a rare moment when we fully get to understand the gifts and full bounty of our earth. Sweetness in our lives often involves processed sugar which is highly addictive, rots teeth, and contributes to the obesity that newspapers scream about. What are we reaping that we have sown? The quality of our nourishment must have diminished if our children are simply getting fat. Although we in more affluent countries may not be actively starving, something in us is not receiving the warm glow of satisfaction acquired from nourishing sustenance. Obsessive "healthy eating" can create its own strange stress.

As the trees lose their leaves so too will we encounter loss on all sorts of levels. How we mourn and grieve our losses has a lot to do with how easily we can negotiate change and find new sources of value all around us. Nature models death with unceasing regularity yet following bereavement and tragedy we often mistake tears and grief for weakness, vulnerability for insipidness, and crying as failure. Plants lose their lives and leaves continuously and most significantly during the autumn but for them losing vibrancy and form is simply part of a great cycle. What have we forgotten along our way? Plant spirits can help us to remember that there is a greater order in the cyclical nature of things.

Our healers strive to approach symptoms with a kind of benign indifference that is not to be confused with a lack of compassion and care. We look instead through the lens of the seasonal elements. Symptoms cannot guide us to the deep root of what is amiss, they are merely the messengers. Any symptomatic approach cannot tell us what the spirit is crying out for. The many people who have studied plant spirit medicine over the years have often found the truth of this to be a penny dropping moment, it makes so much sense.

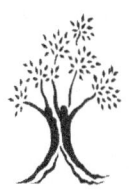

The plant spirit medicine healer doesn't just sit back and observe. What I love about it is the collaboration that happens between myself, the client, the Chinese five elements diagnosis and the plants. The five elements bring our awareness to the rhythms and qualities of each of the seasons, each corresponding to an emotion. The wood element, for example, relates to the spring when the land awakens and the upward rising energy is so strong that we can almost see plants grow. Suddenly we are surrounded with colour, flowers, green, and leaves, so clearly reflected in the times when we feel energy and drive or an upward rising of anger. In autumn, the metal element, the falling leaves teach us how to let go when we grieve a loss or move from one phase of our life on to the next. For me as a PSM healer, it is a continual process of learning how to be with and embody each of the qualities of the elements. How am I with anger, or with joy, how do I receive nourishment, and then let go of things when they are finished? Am I able to rest at the end of it all? I need to be open to touch these places of ease and of discomfort. I am challenged to know myself better so that I may meet my clients in their elemental nature. This inner relationship also opens me to the plants and the natural cycles of the world we live in. **Anna Murray Preece, PSM healer and psychotherapist, UK**

"Ramona" was complaining of a urinary tract infection that got worse when she went on antibiotics. She was in excoriating pain. She had been back to the doctor and received a thorough check-up and everything came out as perfect. But everything wasn't perfect for her. The flare-up had brought intense fear. As the breadwinner, she began to doubt whether she could take care of her family. She had found some symptomatic relief from a naturopath and an acupuncturist, but in her words, they didn't get to what caused it, and she felt worse inside herself. Nobody seemed to help. "It's been an intense five months," she sighed. As I listened I was struck by the paralysing fear that had overtaken her life. I noted the groan in her voice and the smell of a stagnant pond emanating from her body, so I called upon a plant spirit that would restore her waters, bringing calmness and relief to her constant fear. "I feel very relaxed, like I haven't felt in months," she reported after the treatment. "And so spacey, like my mind has turned off." When she came back Ramona reported that it felt like something was moving and shifting, that her resistance was leaving. She no longer felt any separation between work and play. She felt very confident. Over the next few months, Ramona showed signs of improvement in all areas of her life. She no longer had sleep troubles, her fear subsided, and her relationship with her spouse was better than ever. Her gratitude to the plant spirits was equal to mine. **Alison Gayek, PSM healer and senior teacher of PSM, USA**

There have been a few problems for our medicine with the appropriation of the term plant spirit medicine as a generic rather than specific term; one is that the growing popularity of ceremonial use of the sacred plant teachers such as ayahuasca, peyote, and cannabis amongst others has become associated in many people's minds with the medicine we practise; the other is that the greatest strength of PSM—that of its very exact and effective diagnostic and treatment protocols—is not widely understood. It remains a little known modality and one that you can't learn by reading a book. In fact too much head-work is generally a hindrance when it comes to getting into the zone required for connecting with the plants, or to deeply listening with all of the senses to a patient's story, which we do in order to be as accurate as possible in meeting the needs of their spirit.

The plants touch something, chip away at the illness, the dis-ease. They dig something up—this gets pulled out of the person's soul, wherever it is. We have a way of finding it. It is a sort of team effort. Although of course it's the plants who do the actual healing, the healer's job is to identify the need by reading the cries of the spirit correctly. The healing is a mystery, something that can never be fully explained. We can't know how the plants will touch someone, only that they will. We hope that these accounts give a tantalising flavour of our approach, the rigour and science of its protocols, the depth of its reach, and even a taste of the energetic realm it emerges from.

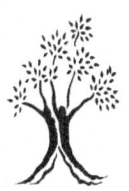

"Deirdre" came to me complaining of mucus building up in her lungs, a chronic problem with repeated lung infections. She understood that something on a deeper level had fallen out of balance. She wanted to see if the plant spirits could release the cause. She reported that during the first treatment she could feel subtle tingling and movement in her chest area. After the treatment she could not feel anything different. However, next morning she realised that she was not coughing at all and her breathing was clear. She felt lighter in herself. Then the realisation "touched me quite deeply" that her father's death anniversary was coming up soon and she had forgotten it. She felt on the verge of tears. She understood that she had to process that loss and her repeated lung infections began to make sense: built-up grief. She was quite emotional. The following day she suddenly became aware that she was also coming up to the anniversary of her sister's death, who had died fifteen years ago in a "devastating accident". Her family had been impacted monumentally but hardly ever talked about it. Deirdre now realised she was carrying so much unexpressed grief. She understood that because it had not been discharged through crying and the whole grieving process, her grief had lodged in her lungs and made her susceptible to infections. She told me, "I love life, life is good, but I've got homework to do." **Dawn Rafferty, PSM healer, Ireland**

Part of what gives the medicine its extraordinary power is knowledge of how various conditions can block or even derail the healing process. These include what are called "outlaw energies" which somehow get into our system and disengage the natural laws making it effectively impossible to bring anything into balance. With the help of our plant allies we can clear these blocks to treatment and understand why nothing seemed to work when they were present in the system of the patient. There are various ways of detecting the presence of these "outlaws".

> One young man was unable to let go of old relationships and felt plagued by grief unspent. He suffered from panic attacks and paranoid thoughts, and while he held down a job, it was a torment to him. He … had experimented quite heavily with Ecstasy and other drugs. When I looked deep into his eyes, I saw a blankness, a lack of response. In Plant Spirit Medicine we call this "possession" and we have a particular plant that knows how to help with it. I was led to ask for assistance from another plant ally by a whiteness I saw in his face and his smell, reminiscent of vitamin pills. This was Snowdrop—a plant of exquisite purity and beauty, which has let me know that it can help people know their own worth, their own purity and goodness. After a few months of PSM the panic attacks had stopped, and after a year he was happy in a new relationship and had found a job that wasn't torture. (Waller, 2018b)

Sometimes we can see the illness leave by signs it makes as it exits. It can happen for instance that short-lived symptoms arise as the deeper issue is working its way out of the very core of our beings. These we call "aggravations", borrowing the observation from homoeopathy's understanding of the way deep healing happens, known as the Law of Cure. Healing crises can be expressed as emotional release, for instance a person may need to cry a lot if there has been a great suppression of grief. Sometimes aggravations are more physical: perhaps a recurrent childhood sore throat that had been repeatedly treated with antibiotics might resurface in order to be cleared from the system. These types of healing reactions are totally normal and indicate that deep healing is taking place. They are transient and will normally last no longer than a day or two. One client reported, "After one treatment I had early on in receiving the medicine I had a really high fever for just 24 hours—it was as if it was an infection, a virus—but there was a lot of people around and nobody else was affected. I just had this huge fever, and the next day it was gone and I felt great."

This isn't to say that every reaction is a sign of healing—sometimes symptoms indicate the need for particular treatment. By following the protocols of the five elements system we seek to accurately track the energetic response of our clients to the effect of the plant spirits. We don't actually know how the healing happens but we do know how to track the movements that are set in motion by their intervention. Thanks to the ancient and sophisticated understanding of the ways in which energy moves through our human systems we can follow the energetic ripples in the wake of the plant spirits' visit.

The art of pulse taking is an invaluable way to directly monitor how a person has received the medicine of the plants. It is possible to feel deeply what is going on within a person by sensitive command of this listening with the fingers. Pulse taking is a rigorous discipline and requires focused, concerted yet simultaneously relaxed concentration. At the same time as having a very elegant yet complex diagnostic methodology and treatment protocol, our medicine also has a magical dimension because it offers a bona fide doorway to the inconceivably rich realm of the plant spirits. It's as if the exacting rigour acts as an anchor in an extraordinary ocean that we can only properly visit with safety and efficacy when we are well and truly held.

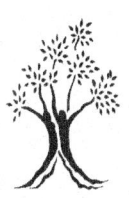

I was finishing my PSM clinicals and we had a healing session with a friend I knew with many health issues and lots of fear and doubt about everything. Her treatment involved many steps. I was still new to the medicine, yet could feel her pulse changes easily and began to see an energetic transformation happening. At the end her face had become uncharacteristically soft and calm. She said she felt at peace. That look of fear and doubt she always had was gone! I commented on this profound shift of energy, countenance, and spirit. My teacher saw it too. All three of us felt the deep release from her chronic fear and doubt. A gift I was humbly able to help with by sharing the medicine of the plant spirits. **K'Anna Burton, PSM healer and SFC fire keeper, USA**

I often find that the plants make themselves known to me just before they are needed ... this was the case with meadowsweet. I decided to journey to it as I came upon a huge field of this beautiful plant. She told me, "I am a balm for the soul, softening the edges of pain and separation. A reminder of the sweetness of original love and innocence, the love you were born in and still dwell in. It's just that you forget ... I will help you remember ...." A short time later I was contacted by a young mother of a two-week-old baby. The baby was having trouble latching on and getting enough milk. I sensed a block in the matriarchal line to do with trust, feeling safe to be fully embodied and that nourishment will be provided. Along with other protocols, meadowsweet was the perfect helper, to restore a trusting in, and receiving of, the sweetness of life. The baby fed well immediately after this treatment, and thanks to the determination of her mother went on to breastfeed very successfully. **Lynn-Amanda Brown, interspecies communicator, creative kinesiologist, and SFC fire keeper, Wales, UK**

As PSM healers our focus is always on the deep call of the spirit as expressed by elemental imbalance. Symptoms are the messengers of this call. It's important not to shoot them and thereby unwittingly contribute to the denial that surrounds our holistic health. Underneath the symptoms are the roots of the imbalance. The plants are compassionate and generous. They are full of love for humans and very willing to share their medicine. Each healer builds a materia medica by making friendships with the plants, not by information someone else gives. It is a living, breathing medicine. There are some plants we all call on in the same kind of way, some that come into every treatment at some point, and others with which we have a very personal and particular connection.

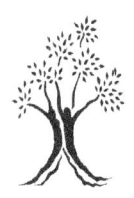

I was driving home from work. My son was very little. I was exhausted. I was doing the course. You've got to do all these journeys, plant studies, somehow fit them in. The meadowsweet was out and it had been waving at me for weeks and I thought right, I'll stop here and hang out with this meadowsweet by the side of the road. I sat there and did a plant study, and it was lovely. Then I journeyed to it there and then, in the car, and when I asked "Is there anything I can do for you?" it said "Go home and have a sleep!" I felt so held by the loving compassion of the meadowsweet who knew my needs better than I was able to know them at that time. **Pip Waller, PSM healer and herbalist, Wales, UK**

I've got a plant that told me it's specifically for men's libido problems. It's a beautiful little plant that grows in the Alps. I had this man who came to me soon after I had met it and amongst other things this was one of his problems, erectile dysfunction I think it's called. After two treatments the problem was completely gone—he was delighted and it transformed his relationship. Since then I've had at least fifteen other men coming with the same thing. The plant told me it's a special remedy for this problem—but you need two sessions! **Lucy Harmer, PSM healer, feng shui and space clearing expert, Switzerland**

An example of what the mind would like to know immediately pops up in relation to this story. "What plant could that be? I want to use it for healing in that way. It could be the new herbal Viagra!" This is not how plant spirit medicine works—remember, a plant offers its medicine to each individual healer differently and based on personal relationship. It's often said that the plants know who will be coming to consult for our help and arrange for us to get to know them accordingly, before the need arises. This is very different from the one-size-fits-all model.

We do, however, have a specific plant for alignment problems. This plant, mugwort, offers wonderful help for our musculoskeletal systems through a simple technique called the "hole in one". Students of the medicine learn this procedure, an adaptation of a chiropractic technique, fairly early on in the training, after appropriate initiation. It brings a great preview of the satisfaction the healer can experience, and is in itself a potent treatment. For instance, one PSM healer treated a person with a severe spinal disc problem that had showed up in an MRI scan as needing an operation. After two hole-in-ones every week for a couple of months another scan showed enormous healing and no need for surgery.

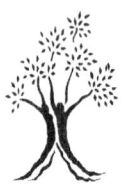

I had this client, she was a pleasure to interview; she'd had so many life experiences. She smoked like a trooper, breathlessness was one of her problems. When she got on the table she started having a massive panic attack. She said, "Everything I've told you, it's all come up and it's a lot." I gave her the hole-in-one treatment and when it was over she said, "Oh my God, that was amazing, the minute you did it my breathing changed." Three years ago she had noticed while meditating that her breathing had changed from her belly to her chest. It returned to her belly right from the start of the treatment. She felt a lot of movement in the abdomen and the hips. She had a very powerful experience from the treatment. When I went to see her about ten days later she was buzzing. Her friends had noticed that her breathing had changed, she wasn't breathless any more. Her posture had changed, she was now sitting up really straight and her smoking had cut in half without her even trying. "It's brilliant. I can breathe again." **Louisa Dix, PSM healer, UK**

"You are totally shattered," she said to me as I stood at her door, she looking at me with wise woman eyes. It wasn't just a bad day. What I had was a sense that my life force had been totally drained out, and it now took extreme effort and pain to deal with ordinary life challenges. If this dark angel has thus far passed you by, it is near impossible to convey effectively the terrible pain of drowning in sorrow, hopelessness, and fearful helplessness when in severe or "clinical" depression. It seemed that every unfairness, disappointment, rejection, inability, betrayal, and abandoned dream I ever experienced decided to gang up on me like a herd of large cats with freshly sharpened claws. They would converge upon me nightly and proceed to tear whatever I had been to shreds.

I couldn't laugh, I couldn't love, I couldn't hope, I couldn't even try anymore. The darkest of angels seeped into the darkest crevices of my soul. Though I had not ever seriously considered this before, the thought of ending my life extended its dark-angel hand towards me offering relief ... and I took great interest. On a dismal night in May, I found the unbearableness too unbearable. I was in my car, and saw myself driving headlong into a concrete embankment. As I scanned the concrete, the vision of a dear acquaintance appeared and somehow I drove to her home instead. I didn't know she did any kind of healing, but she had me lie on a massage table and did some subtle adjustment to my spine and legs. She asked me a question or two. She said that an undisclosed "little plant spirit" was going to "balance my energy". I do not know what happened. I lay there with some hope that I would be lifted up and evaporated and free from this plane and its agony. For twenty-five minutes I lay still. Overall, I could perceive nothing happening, though I did relax. At some point, I felt a very subtle retuning. Then I was beset with total body convulsions, gently twitching on the table for what seemed like a solid minute or two. I looked at her and noticed an involuntary smile creeping over my face for the first time in three months, like a returning dear friend in the distance. I returned home somewhat stabilised, though not sure what, if anything had happened. The most amazing miracle was yet to come. Profound gratitude could be felt moving into my heart, hopes, and organ systems as I drove away and continued to develop over the next week. This was an amazing, long-lasting gratitude high. It hovered around me and in me like a big magic cloud. The pain was not over, but the inclination to take my own life was now quite banished. She was right, you know. I was truly shattered. But instead of depression, I now describe it as a midlife metamorphosis. By the way, the situations that tormented then are still quite present in my life. But now they have no claws, and appear in my mind's eye as dark, silent statues in the deep shadows. Should they animate again, I will not fear them. **Laurie Fisher, fiddler and dance caller, USA**

A decade ago I was having so much difficulty with my back that I could barely walk without excruciating pain. A friend of mine offered me a hole-in-one. What transpired for me was nothing short of opening the floodgates to a new way of being. When I lay down on her table and she put her hands on me I instantly began to cry. I sobbed out loud as my body, my being, shook and

writhed on the table outside time and space. I felt drawn to pursue the plant spirit medicine class for my own personal development, not with the idea that I would "quit my day job". Connecting with the spirit of plants and five elements theory expanded my world-view beyond my greatest imagination! Becoming more and more aware of how much the plants have to offer and their amazing generosity I could not keep this experience to myself. Indeed, I did quit my day job in 2012! Deepening my relationship with the plant world is an ongoing, lifelong learning process that teaches me how to be more in balance with the natural world and myself. Never underestimate the power of a hole-in-one!
Kate Barrier, PSM healer and SFC fire keeper, USA

How we choose the plants to use for a specific person is a mixture of diagnostic art using our exact treatment protocols, and intuition. No two treatments are ever exactly alike even if the same plant spirit is regularly called. No two journeys are the same. The process is incredibly creative and always provides a glimpse of an extraordinarily dynamic world. Although progress may sometimes be slow and not exactly a firework display, nevertheless the smallest shifts towards balance can provide both huge relief and unexpected insights.

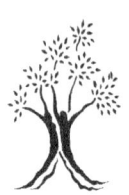

I worked with this gentleman for a year, and he was grey. He had no passion, he was basically one of the walking grey dead people. He was one of those wearing golden handcuffs as they say, which means that he had fallen into middle management in a big corporation and the money was too good and he was stuck. He loved to write but he never gave it any time. He went to work, he made his money, and the benefits were too good to give up. He had prostate issues, blood pressure issues, and was terrified to lose his job, so he put up with being treated poorly, talked badly to. He didn't push back, he had no boundaries. He was just grey. We started working with the plant spirit medicine. Over the course of the year, he started speaking up, "No, not going to do that, no, not working overtime." He carried on working, but he was beginning to dream and he was beginning to write. He started his passion, working on a book. Then he was told he was being laid off—if this had happened a year ago he'd have been destroyed. But by this time, his response was "Good!" He left the job with joy and a good severance package and he wrote his book and it was published. He came to see me and handed me his published book. It was such an amazing day! **Monika Ghent, PSM healer and herbalist, Canada**

One part is going out in nature and creating a relationship and connection to plant spirits and elementals. In my space clearing activities, I work with elementals which are the tiny particles and nature spirits relating to the different elements. When you call them to help you with space clearing they'll come to help out. They can lift, transform, and balance the energy in a space. They can touch every aspect of the essence of a place. In terms of plant spirit medicine it's the same—connecting to the spirits of nature and building relationship with plant spirits. Then figuring out which plant spirit has the right healing energy that a person needs. Sometimes a plant spirit jumps into my mind and goes "Yes, me!" For example I had one woman come to see me who'd had continuous heavy menstrual bleeding for two years. She'd taken all kinds of drugs, hormones, treatments. As she was talking to me about her problem, two plants jumped into my mind. I gave her a PSM treatment (using the five elements protocols) and afterwards as I happened to have these herbs I brewed her a pot of tea. Her periods stopped within an hour and she never had any recurrence. **Lucy Harmer, PSM healer, feng shui and space clearing expert, Switzerland**

Our medicine involves the healer holding a perspective which we call the vision of wholeness. This is the envisioning of what we are, in all our unique beauty, free from the clouds of imbalance that shadow us. It provides a very special blueprint for our potential, a visionary map of how to live optimally. It is not a quick fix nor is it a linear process. Just as plants take time to move through their cycles so does treatment take its time to move and touch us in accordance with multifaceted conditions.

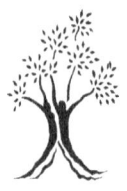

It's so interesting how this medicine works—for me it's more retrospective. I have to look back, then I say, holy crumbs, I'm a totally different person to what I was before! I didn't have anything flashy that suddenly disappeared or anything. It was more subtle, but deeply profound. And I see a lot of that in my practice. You have to commit to ten treatments before you can make any judgement about the medicine—this is no quick fix, this medicine. There are things that instantly clear up for sure—you may have a headache and it's gone, or an anxiety, and it's gone, this can be quick. But that's like anything—herbal medicine, or taking an aspirin even. It's not the real healing, it's just symptomatic, and this is not a symptomatic medicine. **Monika Ghent, PSM healer and herbalist, Canada**

The concept of "curing disease" results from a medical science approach to ailments through medication and external intervention, which is great for broken bones, or those hopefully rare instances in our lives when we need surgery. But physical symptoms of "dis-ease", especially chronic symptoms, often result from spiritual imbalance that can only be alleviated through an approach to healing the spirit. Plant spirit medicine will not cure, but most certainly will invite healing. Healing can mean you learn to forgive yourself, and thereby forge new relationships with the natural world as it upholds and relates and connects with your inner world, including all of those things "ailing" you. Why is one treatment not enough? As a healer in this modality, I need to get to know you, more as a friend than a client, because when we begin treatment I need to introduce you to my plant friends. I need to show them I know you in a way they can understand and relate to, so that they can help you. Getting to know each other takes time. You might feel better after one treatment, but only after repetition of going out into the world, coming back to the plants, then going back into your life can there be a foundation for you to maintain this new balance that is taking hold. This allows me to see how your outer life impacts your inner balance so I can properly communicate this to the plant spirits that will help you. **Buffy Aakaash, PSM healer and SFC fire keeper, USA**

> *You might like to now repeat the exercise suggested in Chapter 1 of sitting with a plant with a view to getting to know it, this time with the addition of making an offering. Prepare your offering of barley or oatseed if you are in Europe, or tobacco if you are in the Americas. Follow the instructions for the exercise on p. 7, this time introducing yourself out loud by name and giving the plant your offering (literally sprinkle it on or near the growing plants). See how this act of exchange affects your experience.*

The principle of exchange inherent in the indigenous perspective has for so long been replaced in our culture by a consumerist mindset that we are rarely even aware of how much we simply take. Relationship and exchange with our generous plant allies is at the heart of our practice of the medicine. When we sit with a plant to begin to get to know it, we offer barley, oats, or tobacco as a token of our willingness to be part of this great web, an acknowledgement that for all we receive, we are happy to give.

We may also ask the plants who become our allies in this way if they require anything from us in exchange for gifting our people with their medicine. As part of our training we are initiated into the use of certain plant spirits and given guidance by them as to what might be required of us in order to proceed. We don't name all the plants because we're not hostages to our mind's insatiable demand for factual information which it claims as real knowledge. This is likely to stir up resistance in the form of mental frustration. Good! This is part of the process required for a paradigm shift.

It's not that plant spirit medicine is effective in every circumstance. For example, it can't put right a problem that comes from breaking a sacred law. The story on p. 17 about Sameera and the rock she took from an Aboriginal sacred site illustrates one such problem. Another problem could be the misuse of sacred plant teachers which in themselves are a type of spiritual doorway. Sometimes another kind of healing is required.

There is something mysteriously different about the practice of plant spirit medicine as compared to other natural medicine modalities. It's not easy to pin down. We don't really know what the plant spirits are up to. We don't know what effect they'll have, how their medicine will play out in a person's life. The medicine is not in any way symptomatic, it's not about us needing to understand symptoms and match them with a medicine. It's not about us figuring out with the patient their wounds, where they need to work, and then asking the plants to help with that. Although this does naturally happen as part of the rapport-building relationship, and is a very beautiful and nourishing part of the therapeutic relationship, it's not the core of PSM. This part of the therapy is a part of what we as *human* healers are endeavouring to provide. Yet the vast and mysterious power of the realm of the plant spirits is beyond anything our humans minds can fully recognise or pin down. In plant spirit medicine you are not a practitioner, you are a healer, a friend of the plants who are the divine healers.

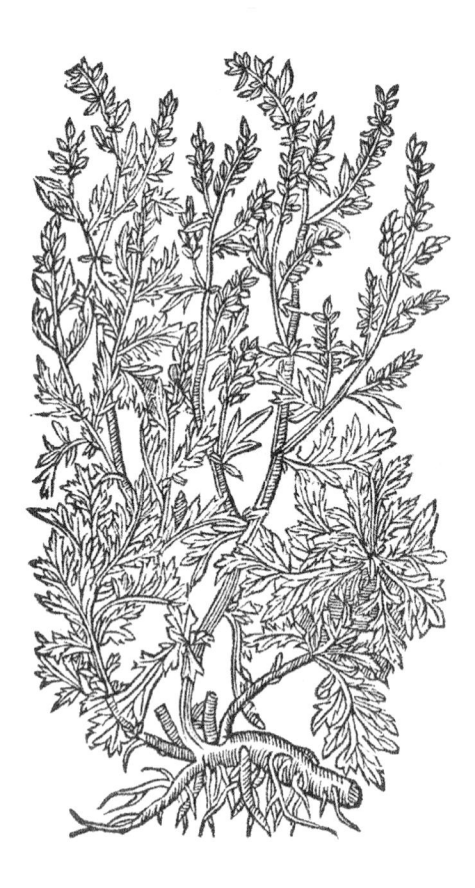

Mugwort from Parkinson's Herbarium.

CHAPTER THREE

Receiving the medicine

I am writing to thank you for whatever magic you worked earlier in the year. I was in a poor way, the colour had gone along with my joy for life. Looking back I have no doubt I was descending into depression. A work client was concerned and paid for me to have a consultation with you. You listened to my story from beginning to end, properly and deeply, giving me all the time I needed. After your treatment I left feeling tangibly different. Very hungry actually and, unusually, took myself to bed with a hot-water bottle in the afternoon. The next day I woke feeling entirely back to normal! It felt like the missing brick in my foundations had been booted back into place. It was quite extraordinary and I have no doubt you saved me from a long dark journey. I haven't looked back since.

This chapter attempts to show something of the experience of receiving the medicine of the plant spirits by using first-person accounts in patients' own words, and interesting case histories. We want the effects of the plant spirits' healing to speak for itself. The stories demonstrate the irrepressible fusion of the down to earth with the totally inexplicable and miraculous that the medicine of the plants has to offer. While many come from plant spirit medicine healers in our own tradition, these offerings include experiences from other approaches to healing with plant spirit or plant energy. All the stories in this chapter are anonymous to protect patients' privacy.

The best thing for me about receiving plant spirit medicine has been how it has helped me reconnect to the plants and their love. It has been like a homecoming and has opened many doors ... as well as the immediate relief of feeling back in balance physically and emotionally after a treatment.

What ails us?

If we look at the way we are living through the lens of the cycle of the seasons it isn't hard to see how far from a natural approach we have come. We are now mostly living in urban or otherwise compromised environments where it might feel very difficult to know what is happening in the world of nature, let alone return to it. But however much our lives may be enveloped in concrete, tarmac, money, and consumption, we are still living under a sky and standing on the earth, with sunlight falling, and growing, moon and stars appearing out of darkness in patterns beyond our ken. We remain subject to disease however much we cut, reduce, analyse, colonise, name, measure, or develop the science of rockets or artificial intelligence. We are born and we die. The simplicity of this orientation could be criticised in our supposedly highly evolved world, but within simplicity is the elegance of complexity unravelled. Nothing could be more complex than nature's limitless creative possibilities, and still the plant spirits are simply offering us their help. Perhaps what is really making us sick is that we have forgotten our place in the grand scheme, we've been so busy grabbing and competing. As the poet Wordsworth wrote in the nineteenth century, "Getting and spending we lay waste our powers."

In a world of imbalance, how can we help being off kilter ourselves? The cry of our spirit may come as physical symptoms, ailments and diseases, mental anguish, emotional need, or spiritual hunger. Even when the cry screams inside us, still it is often much quieter than the noisy, busy world we inhabit. It is part of the invisible that we are so keen to ignore due to its lack of material substance, and yet it is constant. It is made up of histories and hurts, of traumas and undisclosed pain, of confusion, misunderstanding, mistakes, and lack of learning. It often feels old yet keeps being born, gets recreated in families manifesting in a myriad of illnesses that further perpetuate tragedy and sorrow. It is depression, suicide, self-harm, sickness, addiction, oppression, violence, pain, and deadly boredom. It is gruelling cancer, road traffic accidents, child abuse, isolation, poverty, loneliness, theft, and rape. It is a feeling of numbness or emptiness, a hole that cannot be filled. It is ultimately total disconnection, not just from each other and the world, but from our own selves. Or it might simply be a feeling that something is amiss, just not quite right inside. Internal feeling is quiet and personal. Sadly, spiritual malaise is so commonplace we think it's the way life should be. We've got used to it as a way of life. People seek out healing for all these many reasons, and more. The following stories are a patchwork of the plants' answers to our cries, and the unforeseeable way they facilitate change.

I was three years into the menopause, experiencing the classic symptoms of hot flushes, night sweats, mood swings, chronic insomnia, and depression. What I did not expect was a return of acute eczema symptoms, a lifelong condition that had been in abeyance for a number of years, but now leaving me feeling utterly wretched. My expectation was to see an immediate improvement as I had taken a sabbatical year (I teach the Alexander Technique and meditation, one to one, in groups and workshops). Who knew I would become so ill and depressed to the point of not wanting to remain in this body? In my desperation, I contacted a local shaman healer, suspecting these symptoms were a part of something ancestral, as all treatments I tried were palliative only and could not prevent this onslaught of severe burning, itching, and tearing apart my poor body. The healer recommended my local plant spirit medicine healer. I was intrigued to find out more online while waiting for my first appointment.

The most profound statement made during my first session was not to ask the question "why" I was unwell, rather to trust the plants to guide me through the doorway into another set of possibilities. And so the healing work began. It hasn't been a miracle cure but, for me, it has been miraculous. After twelve months of regular sessions, my body is beginning to recover ever so slowly. I am less frequently on fire, my skin is almost its normal colour, less chronically dry and itchy. I am less irritable, scratch much less, and am sleeping a lot better. Dreaming has begun its long awaited return, albeit sporadically, along with yawning and stretching, things I never thought I would miss. The plant spirits are teaching me patience, and to not expect. The natural outcome of that is to be present, alert to what is. My sessions continue. I no longer look for outcomes as I am experiencing a total different way of connecting to my environment. There have been intense moments of joy in my heart for this life, gratitude for all that I have, and all that is being revealed to me though the work of the plants. After such a long time feeling helpless and at the mercy of this illness, I am finally coming into the light.

Receiving the spirit medicine of the plants completely reoriented my life and helped me to see that I wasn't on the outside of nature looking at it, but a part of it. Though I sometimes forget this, it helps me remember that everything in existence is somehow connected: rocks, dead wood, water, and such things we often pass off as inert objects. This deep connection also made me occasionally cynical of the cold, always calculating world we live in. Feeling cynicism is a sign for me that I need a treatment with the plant spirits, because the plants are not at all cynical. If humans were to fail to survive, I'm quite certain the plants would rebound, because after millions of years of growing and evolving they understand how to survive, which is through community. I've always been drawn to the topic of community, and the plants helped me to understand how crucial it is in order to thrive.

I was introduced to plant spirit medicine by a close friend who thought it could help me recover from a particularly bad bout of pneumonia which had me hospitalised and had really taken its toll on my energy and ability to recover. I had used herbalism before but was not au fait with this spiritual type of plant healing. However, I was open to the idea and trusted my friend's judgement. I found it very easy to relate to my healer. She didn't extol the virtues of her beliefs or wax lyrical about how plant spirit medicine works. She listened, coaxed answers to pertinent questions about life events prior to getting sick, as well as taking a general health history. During the treatment I became overwhelmed by emotion. Tears welled up and I felt incredible sadness with a powerful sense of loss, mingled with anger and resentment. With gentleness and compassion I was advised total rest for at least a couple of days. Thus started what has now been an ongoing journey. I have no idea how it works—all I know is that since I started, I have had far fewer infections especially of the chest, and if I do get ill, I recover much more quickly than before. I have let go of emotions bound up with loss and resentment and anger, which I really did think I had dealt with, but obviously hadn't. I have long known about and been interested in the interconnectedness of everything and am aware of both scientific and spiritual approaches to understanding and experiencing this. I love the natural world and have enjoyed helping to create a garden and a woodland so am aware of the beauty and power of plants. However, I have now also experienced the plant spirit medicine way of healing whereby a healer with certain knowledge and experience can use plants in a particular way combined with the dynamic which occurs in a good relationship with the client.

I was always tormented, really, by a lack of self-esteem and value for my own self. No matter what I accomplished, what I did, nothing would ever touch the feeling that I wasn't enough, I wasn't good enough, I wasn't doing enough, I had to do better. And it haunted me—it was a haunting. I'd been haunted by this forever, and nothing touched it. But since I've been receiving healing from the plant spirits I don't have that any more. I can't tell you what that is worth to me. I still have times of feeling incredibly humbled and feeling that I could have done better at something, or like I want to do better in my relationship with someone, but it's not the same way. It's from a place of strength, it's actually healthy, to have a healthy sense of humbleness that is good. I'd say I'm humble, but not ashamed. This has changed me. It's given me courage to do things, to hear my heart voice so I know I'm on the right path, the right direction. I can hear my inner guidance, I can hear the guidance of great spirit. So it's changed my whole life—it's been amazing. When I received the medicine, the first time the plant spirits touched me, I was riddled with grief and I cried and cried. Through the whole treatment I cried and I could actually smell a plant that I knew was used for grief: it was wild ginger. I smelt it during my treatment and I was crying. I sat up with my bloodshot eyes and my wet face and I said, wow, there's a lot of grief in my body! The healer just looked at me and said "Aha!" (they never tell you anything). I get a treatment at least every month. I can't go too long without having a treatment, I feel it's so nourishing. It makes me feel so grounded and present, I am committed to this medicine completely—it's cradle to the grave medicine—and on my last dying breath I'll be getting a treatment for sure because it does so much for me!

I sought out help from the plant spirits at an extremely low point in my life. I was financially, physically, spiritually, and morally bankrupt. I had bottomed out on alcohol and drugs, my business had evaporated, I had been largely abandoned by friends and especially family and was living in fear of the future. I was attracted to plant spirit medicine because people to whom I was close, some of the few people that had not given up on me, were both receivers and practitioners of the medicine. They had what I wanted, an inner serenity and clarity I had seldom seen that was unmoved by externals; a solid core that I was well aware I lacked. Over time, with regular treatments, I have grown tremendously, and while, like all of us, I will always have further to go I am at a place of peace with my life, despite it being difficult in some ways. I have accepted my family's inability to form loving bonds and their narcissistic fixation on appearance over substance. I am less trapped in the hedonistic treadmill of financial striving and I have gained the ability to form real, lasting bonds with others based on a spiritual connection rather than competitive social striving. I have also become open to the pursuit of a spiritual path that both challenges and soothes me. To the curious, I would say to let down your guard and be open to the great mystery. We do not have to understand a spiritual path to grow from its pursuit.

One woman made an appointment. I open the door and she's not even standing at my door, she's down the walkway. She comes in, gives a perfunctory "Hello", brushes by me, and goes into the office. She was an extremely guarded person, not chatty, didn't have any kind of laughter or anything. She was closed and allergic to everything, couldn't handle the world. She had to wear a scarf around her neck when she went anywhere. She seemed kind of bitter, couldn't stand anything, and people bugged her. We started working with the plant spirits and although it took a while, she totally changed. Over time, she came alive. Now she is funny and witty and warm. She doesn't freak out about going into public, she's not guarded, she's her own person, she has what she needs to be OK. As she walks through the world she's no longer affected nor allergic in that way she was. Her whole life changed, she is sparkly and alive, so engaged.

I've led a full life, my life. I was brought up typical working class council estate, rough and tumble. As a child I had constantly grazed knees from playing on my skateboard and making dens, that kind of thing. From there I started a drinking career from the early age of fourteen or fifteen. This was my downfall. It had a hold of me, due to my life experience. I carried on drinking until the age of thirty-eight, then I got to the jumping off place, sick of being sick. I joined AA and it opened the door to me having an understanding of spirituality and an openness to different types of healing treatments. I'd heard it said how emotions play a role in life and how stuck emotions can make people poorly, so I was happy to go ahead with this plant spirit medicine and whatever it held for me. I felt I had nothing to lose. So there I am having my treatments, and it's just wonderful to have a healer who's someone I can talk to in a safe environment. That in this modern age is quite priceless. So when I receive my healing we talk, and then I lie on the treatment couch, she takes my pulses. Once I lie on that bed there's this peace every time that comes over. I am so relaxed, knowing I'm being taken care of, someone is there, healing me the way these PSM healers heal, and it's wonderful. I always end up leaving a treatment feeling different. More energised, more loving, I feel the balance. This is what I've yearned for all the way through my life—physical balance, emotional balance, spiritual balance. Until now I'd led a life of imbalance.

Receiving the medicine of plant spirits has brought understanding to me. One is the word *spirit*. Two, is Mother Nature. I have got a bounty of love now for Mother Nature. I think of mother and I can feel my heart beat and this feeling of intense unconditional love comes over me, and I could shed a tear. And this I never had before. Then there's spirit—an understanding of spirit in plants, trees, everywhere. There's a wholeness, we're all attached, the plants and Mother Nature are just there and they give freely. I've been living my life like this for a couple of years now and I've come to realise that there's an attitude of gratitude. So when I go on my daily walk I have a pocketful of barley, and if I connect, or if I don't connect, with a tree, I will still be making offerings that day, to Mother Nature, to the plants. And it's a wonderful way; it's my way of saying thanks to nature. My life has been so much better since I've been receiving plant spirit medicine.

Since beginning treatment, there has been a profound shift in my artistic practice. Something has fallen into place at a fundamental level. I am connecting with audiences in a much deeper way. I have had people say that my storytelling feels deeply grounded; that through my telling of stories they also feel connected. They have phrased what they are connected to differently—to the past, to the land, to a sense of belonging, to an ongoing tradition, but they feel a connection through the stories. I have always loved traditional British stories; their power and magic, the wealth of knowledge and memory that they carry ... but I could never quite convey the same power and beauty on my tongue that they had in my heart. That seems to be changing. The sacred fire (see p. 144 and 166) has also had a huge impact on my storytelling. Any new big piece I work on, I now tell to the fire first. The first time I did this, I wasn't prepared for how it would feel. I thought it would be rather lovely, with an understanding, friendly audience. Rather unexpectedly, it felt more like (and was) trial by fire! But it worked. The fire burned away extraneous rubbish and got to the heart of what needed to happen. It has been a slow and subtle process, but looking back to where I was two and a half years ago, I am so much more comfortable and confident as an artist—and really excited by the creative opportunities that have opened up before me.

My son was about fourteen months old and had never slept all night. After my first plant spirit medicine treatment he immediately started sleeping through. It was a lifesaver. At that time I was very depleted from continual lack of sleep and the treatment restored me. I didn't have a lot of physical problems except for that but I feel like what the plants did for me was bring me home to myself so I could focus on what was important in life. They made all of my life richer; relationships, things I was pursuing, all the important things. There's a lot of what we "should do" in life, and a lot of Western culture values that weren't my values, so it brought me back to what was really right for me.

I entered the treatment room not knowing what to expect. Although I had been swept along I didn't really know what a treatment might entail. I sat for a long time completely tongue-tied. Unable to speak, my heart was pounding in my ribcage and the room appeared to recede from view. A huge sorrow swept up and over me as a wave of memory brought my learning disabled uncle into my awareness. I had not thought or even considered him for the years since he had died and now his experiences appeared to be a tragedy of incredible proportion. Isolated from our family by the breakdown of my parents' marriage he had lost his connection with the sister-in-law he had loved and all his nephews and nieces, whose lives had complemented his simple one with love and a sense of belonging. Nobody had thought to contain him during the explosive break-up, he was visited as a duty but was subsequently institutionalised and thereby lost his meaning and we lost him and his uncomplicated dedication. That day I was able to contact the full force of shame and sorrow that hitherto had been an unconscious quiet depression held somewhere in my being and start to properly grieve.

This story is to do with rose. This was an experience of somebody with severe endometriosis. After working with her a while we found that her body was holding an incredible degree of trauma that was related to very early heart surgery (as a small child). What transpired was that there was a complete disconnect and even almost a hatred or disgust at her own heart. Somehow this whole medicalisation of that process had profoundly disconnected her from her own heart. I think over many years, and through a lot of work with hawthorn as well, she finally came to a place where she was able to say that she feels like she likes her own heart. That felt like an immense threshold to move through and I feel sure that it wouldn't have been possible without the plants. There's something to do with an acceptance and a gentleness and love, self-love. It's almost like the plants have been whispering these possibilities over years and years and years, and then at some point there's a critical mass: these presences show that they have some kin to this person's being and something is fundamentally changed.

The efficacy of plant spirit medicine defies belief! I am a natural sceptic and never expect to feel anything, and although I do have in some cases a profound experience it always surprises me. I'd like to share an experience I had after receiving healing from the plant spirits. One of the things I always had problems with, due to multiple issues with food allergies and intolerances, was breathing out of my left nostril when lying on my right side in bed at night. I could only lay on the right side for a few seconds and only then if I put pressure on the top of my nose to keep the airway open. As soon as I would fall asleep and my hand relaxed I would wake up and have to turn over because I couldn't breathe properly. I had a session and as usual didn't expect anything to happen. That night I went to bed and spent my usual few minutes on my right hand side before turning onto my left to sleep. I woke up and thought what a wonderful night's sleep I'd had. I didn't rise straight away and as I was lying there I suddenly realised that I had woken up on my right side and was freely breathing through both nostrils—including the left which had been permanently blocked for years. I hadn't been able to breathe when lying on my right side for at least two years that I remember, possibly a lot longer than that! Each time my nose makes breathing difficult I have a treatment and am able to breathe again. I give thanks to plant spirit medicine for the wonderful healing and the amazing effects it has on my physical symptoms and also my heart!

In January 2016 (at age twenty-five) I got diagnosed with pancreas cancer. The doctors told me that I would die within the next six months. They wanted to do chemotherapy even though they thought it wouldn't work. I had had cancer at the age of nine and for a few years had a lot of conventional treatment, and I just didn't want to do chemotherapy this time—but I was determined not to die!

Unfortunately the cancer spread quickly, and soon I was faced with seven tumours. Still I'd never give up. The doctors said there was no chance that I would live, they just saw the end—so I needed alternatives, and healers who would believe in me. I heard about hemp oil and how it could heal people from cancer, and I began the therapy. Within the next eight months, five of the seven tumours disappeared, but still I had tumours in both of my breasts. This was the time when I got my first PSM healing. It felt like medicine growing inside of me, like it was manifesting inside me. A month later I felt empowered and more and more myself again. I stopped using the hemp because I no longer felt it was good for me, even though a scan showed the breast tumours still there. I then had twelve days of intensive healing with plant spirit medicine every day, and everything changed in that time. My inner peace and my happiness found their way back to me, but not just that. Four days after I arrived back home, I had a screening again and all my cancer was gone. Today it's March 2018 and I'm still healthy and happy because I found my way, plant spirit medicine. Thank you from all that I am.

I had pains in my joints, especially my hands. I also experienced other pains that the doctors were unable to identify. The pains seemed to be related to hormones. I had several blood tests and X-rays done but the doctors weren't able to tell what could be causing the symptoms. So I came for help from the plant spirits. My healer is lovely and personable with great knowledge and I felt very comfortable. During the treatments, I felt very relaxed and able to release tension in my mind and body, feelings of being cleansed and coming more into my natural state of being. It has been and is a process where I feel that the plant spirit medicine is supporting my natural growth and assisting my body's own healing process. Now about ten months later the pains I had in my body have diminished. I am less afraid of the symptoms and better notice how my diet and ways of living are affecting my body and mind. The plant spirit medicine treatments seem to be integrating the energy in my body in a way that everything flows better. This gives me the energy and courage to make necessary changes to help me feel better.

As an only child living with four adults I was encouraged to spend as much time as possible in the garden—for which I am very grateful on many levels. I don't recall how old I was when I first noticed the small people in the garden with me. To begin with I caught glimpses of movement at the corner of my eye but gradually figures showed themselves more fully and I would chatter away to them as I played. I remember being vaguely surprised that they were not the delicate, ethereal creatures of my fairy story books but sturdy, rumbustious individuals with a great sense of fun. Of course, when I described my companions to adults I was initially humoured, but as I grew older and persisted with my stories I was reprimanded for telling lies. Despite the disapproval, I continued to catch glimpses of these people in other settings during my life, but it was when I first experienced healing from plant spirits that they came back to me in strength. From the moment I lay on the couch the familiar sense of seeing someone from the corner of my eye began and soon there were dozens of these beings, laughing and dancing around with evident glee. I had a strong sense of "coming home" and feeling recognised. I have experienced a number of interesting sensations where the small people have been working on me. One example that made me laugh was when they got involved with a stubbornly chronic shoulder problem. In the session I was aware of four of the "helpers" standing by my right hand. They rolled up their sleeves and grabbed hold of my middle finger as if to get ready for a tug of war and that is what transpired—they tugged and hauled at something long and sinewy which emerged from my finger. I could distinctly feel the pulling sensation and was highly entertained by the behaviour of the helpers who fell over several times and roared with laughter. Following that session my shoulder made a considerable improvement. On another occasion the small people seemed more subdued and stayed in the background as if on their best behaviour and I became aware of a few, much taller beings who were dressed differently and appeared more serious. The small people appeared slightly in awe of these new individuals and so was I! I wasn't completely sure what they were doing but I felt that they were exerting a strong benevolent influence on me. I asked my healer if she was doing something different this time and she replied that she had called on a different plant spirit helper. When I have plucked up courage to tell friends about my experiences I am pleasantly surprised that so many respond with, "I'm so glad you told me that, I thought it sounded a bit odd but I've seen little beings like that too."

I've been having treatments for many years and it has had a very deep effect on my life. I feel more balanced on many levels; I no longer suffer with chronic bowel problems; very rarely have asthma; my energy levels are much better (looking back my energy was very depleted). And it goes beyond these physical problems. I've always loved being in nature, but the love and respect has deepened and I feel more open now to receive, I feel grounded, more alive and awake. I have a real sense of peace especially when I'm close to trees and plants, the elements. I always had this feeling that I didn't quite belong, maybe I was born in the wrong century or land, like a yearning for something, but I don't feel this any more. After I've had my treatment I usually walk into the town and I have this tremendous sense of connection. I see people in a different light, like my heart is open to everything … I really like this feeling. I've also had other help from the plants. One night my youngest child was having trouble with her asthma, her medication wasn't helping her symptoms, I was in despair, so in my mind I started to scan my garden for a plant to help her. I just couldn't find anything there but I was led to the garden nursery down the road, which I'd been to that day and was looking at lungwort. I spoke with lungwort in my heart, had an exchange with it and asked it to help. My daughter's breathing got easier—I feel the plant really helped us get through the night. I know my healing is a long journey and I feel blessed that I've found this wonderful powerful medicine. It's made me feel more at home with myself and the world, understanding what I need to do to feel balanced and well.

One woman came with a bladder weakness, a mild incontinence. She'd had to start to wear pads. She came for a number of treatments but within a few days of the first treatment her incontinence problem had sorted itself out.

The other amazing thing was, she started to wear brightly coloured clothes. Before that she'd always worn navy or black, plain and smart clothes. There was a whole transformation of her persona. She felt she'd found her real self, like a butterfly emerged from a chrysalis. She'd let go of fears and family issues and found her true self. This ended up more important to her than the incontinence. She was very pleased she'd come for so many sessions. She still comes a couple times a year for her "plein de lumière"—her "fill of light".

An amazing man who couldn't figure out at all what was right for him, what was good for him, and what wasn't good for him, came for treatment. He had explanations that were so lyrical about both sides of an issue, but he couldn't figure out what was good for him. He would talk and go on and on, so rational on both sides, but he was stuck—stuck, stuck, stuck. So the plant spirits gave their medicine, and within a few months his understanding of what he needed became crystal clear, he became able to take things on and knew they were right for him.

"Ann" greeted me in a whisper at the door. I could barely hear her speaking while she told me a story about an abusive relationship she had stayed in for many years. She said, "I was petrified of him." She eventually got out of the relationship a few years before coming to me for help. She told me, "I used to have great clarity of how to live my life. I had a successful business and was always very resourceful for new ideas. Now I can't see anything through. I am even having communication difficulties. It's getting more intense. It's really hard to explain. I am not able to make money. I am walking around in this chaos. I feel like my life is coming to an end, like a car will knock me down or something. I'm just existing, taking up food and air." I called on a plant spirit to restore her boundaries which had been systematically seriously violated. She had been too petrified to express her anger to restore her boundaries. So she was carrying a lot of suppressed rage. She had lost her vitality, her ability to grow and make decisions, focus, and direction. As she left my treatment room she was still barely audible. She had felt nothing worth mentioning in the treatment session. After three days we spoke on the telephone. Her voice was strong. She said that the morning after the treatment she'd felt very focused and peaceful and knew what she wanted to do. She said this felt really great; it was like her direction had returned. She also reported that she had got really angry on the third day. She said, "This happens sometimes, it's like I have no control over it." She felt very ashamed of that. You see, anger motivates us to set up proper boundaries. That's anger's job. When anger becomes dammed up it becomes a problem. Then instead of leading us to set healthy, beneficial boundaries, anger can be distorted to aggression or verbal explosions, or as in her case, a loss of zest for life with the odd isolated, out of proportion explosion.

I am battling a serious long term illness. Treatment by a plant spirit medicine healer gives me a better quality of life and keeps me positive. My energy is better and my vitality stronger. I feel more balanced. I am sure the plant's healing keeps the illness from progressing and helps me live with it without giving in, enabling me to carry on with and enjoy my life.

As I drop to deeper and deeper layers that need healing, I arrive at blocks that are like the tough skins that sometimes occur inside the onion. Subtler means are required to let go of these blocks and for this deeper healing to occur. It has always been at times of need in my own healing journey that life has placed another teacher or healer in my path. Understanding what level of balancing in the being is needed, and where, is for me a major key for healing to take place, and this is often only understood in retrospect.

Although our focus is on medicine for our fellow humans, in fact it's not only people who are helped by the plants. Some healers working with plant spirits also offer healing to animals, and sometimes it's the animals themselves who bring people into the medicine as if they were in league with the plants.

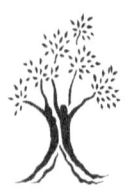

I started working with animals when my own beloved cat, Gwilym, became sick, and I couldn't find anyone who could help him. I read some books on animal communication and it sounded similar to my experiences with plants, so in desperation I gave it a go. Gwilym was very encouraging. After this experience I went on to train with a couple of other animal communicators and combined their teaching with my other healing modalities. I find animals are very receptive to the plants. What follows is a story from a dog owner about one of my clients, a black Labrador cross named Siddhartha Raven Hound—aka Sid.

"I first encountered Sid when I was a volunteer dog walker at a rescue centre near Malvern. I rarely walked Sid because he was so incredibly strong. Sometimes when Sid played alone in a pen I would look at him through the fence. He was such a beautiful dog. He would come over and push his face up close against the fence. After a few weeks of meeting Sid like this I was allowed into the pen to play with him. He was such fun and a very loving dog. We would play with a tennis ball for ages, then sit on the floor of the pen and snuggle up together. One day, I was shocked to learn that the centre had put another dog to sleep for biting a volunteer. From that point on, my husband and I together took Sid for his walks, and I continued to play with him in the pen. One day when Sid was being wound up by a dog in the next pen, he got in a frenzy and bit my hand. He was taken and put in an isolation cage. I was terrified he would be destroyed. We decided to apply to foster Sid. He was kept in isolation until we were ready to take him home. When he finally came to stay with us, it was a dream. He was a great companion in the house, but taking him out was a different matter. He pulled and pulled on the lead, he was so strong. Every dog that passed by, he reacted to. If a man passed by with a stick, Sid went into a frenzy, barking like mad. We were that nervous we would hide behind bushes or walk in the opposite direction any time someone passed by, with or without a dog. We were advised to take Sid to a dog behaviorist, then I remembered that a friend was an animal healer, so I contacted her and asked for help. Within a day, after one distance healing session, Sid was calmer on his walks, and so were we! Every day he improved, until one day we trusted it would be safe to let him off the lead. And sure enough, he was fine and since then we've had no problems with other dogs

RECEIVING THE MEDICINE 57

To do this exercise you will need to find a place where there are a few small plants growing as well as some trees, perhaps somewhere where there are some very different areas, and it is best done at a time of year when the flowers are out. If you don't have access to wild nature then go to a park. Before you arrive, notice how you feel—do a check of your body and emotions, the kind of thoughts you are having. Then find a place where there are trees growing and sit or walk among them for ten minutes or so. Notice any changes in your feelings. Then go to a very different area, where there are smaller plants growing, say a rose garden or buttercup meadow, a patch of nettles or a flower bed. Again spend ten minutes or so among them, noticing how it feels. Return to the trees again and repeat the exercise, comparing the feeling of being around trees with the feeling of being with the herbaceous plants you found. Go between the two as many times as you wish to get a clear sense of this. Try it wherever you are when you get a chance to check in with the "energy" of a different kind of habitat: small sea plants, moorland grasses, a fruit orchard, a beech wood compared with an oak wood, a sea of bluebells, the first snowdrops.

or people." **Lynn-Amanda Brown, interspecies communicator, creative kinesiologist and SFC fire keeper, Wales, UK**

I came across PSM in 2007 when Lucy brought her dog Ruby to see me with an injured hind leg for acupuncture, one of the therapies I use in my integrated holistic veterinary practice. I was checking her pulses according to the five elements Chinese theory when Lucy asked me what I was doing. We started to talk about the different alternative therapies and as destiny would have it, a PSM course was to be held in the UK only a couple of hours away from home, and I embarked on a course that I thought would consolidate my knowledge but in fact opened the door into a whole new world. With thanks to Ruby. **Barbara Jones, holistic vet, UK**

The stories show really clearly the great variety of healing that the plant spirits offer. To get a taste of this diversity, you might like to try the exercise to the left.

Receiving the medicine of the plant spirits spans the mundane to the sublime, and can even make you rich, though we are still working on the winning lottery numbers!

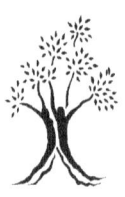

One time I was tidying up in the fire pit in Cornwall. We lived in the dunes so the pit was in sand, surrounded by wild rose and sea buckthorn. Stacking up the chairs I noticed a small flower that had moved into the circle around the hearth. I hadn't seen it there before and on closer inspection I could see it was stork's bill. I was just dusting the sand from its leaves when I felt the edge of something folded up and tucked beneath it. It was a crisp £10 note. Most welcome!

An amazing thing happened one day in my clinic. After leaving a plant spirit medicine session a patient was walking down the street and looked up to admire a beautiful hawthorn tree that grows on the pavement nearby. What should she see but a £5 note! She felt it was a present from the tree as she was worried about money. What makes this even more wonderful is that it was the tree whose spirit was called in to help her in that session.

Joking aside, the signature of the way the plant spirits move in our lives consistently reveals something that goes far beyond help for whatever we thought our problem was in the first place. There is an alignment with the flow and purpose of our lives that is beyond any ability of either healer or patient to foresee. The plants somehow appear to act as matchmakers, estate agents, personnel recruitment officers, spiritual signposts, and more. Time and time again, we witness the pieces of a person's life rearranging. As long as we are willing to commit to the healing process, the plants will bring us not necessarily what our minds tell us we want, but always what we truly need.

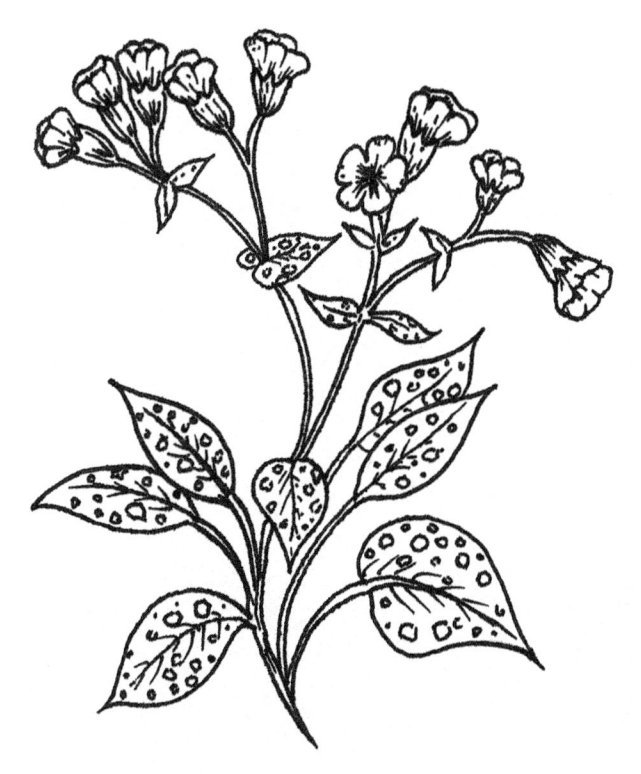

Lungwort by Rachel Lloyd.

CHAPTER FOUR

The journey of the seasons

The plants are calling us to enter the dream of nature. This is a realm far removed from the mental level that modern life compels us to dwell in, yet it is present everywhere that nature resides. Dandelions growing up through cracks in pavements hint at it, the wind carries its whispers, trees in city parks carry its songs. Plant spirit medicine itself arises from this dream and we are its eyes and hands. We are in its service.

One of the most difficult and important challenges for the healer is to correctly diagnose problems in order to be led to the right remedy. The five elements model used by classical plant spirit medicine is really a living representation of the natural world as experienced through the seasons. The elements, being great cosmic energies which move through the world creating all the expressions of life, exist everywhere, in all climates. But it's easiest to get the feeling for them in the context of the temperate zone seasons. We need to feel the seasonal energies, not think about them. We need to dream with them, experience them at the level of our hearts.

Inquiry
The roots,
Traveling unmapped roads
Below,

Or the boughs,
Penetrating the hallways of sky
With each new fistful
Of leaf and bloom?

The chocolate secret realm
Of incubation,
Or the airy rooms
Of unlimited potential?

The seed,
Or the song of the seed in the world?

Louise Berliner (2011)

So what *is* the dream of nature? "Without doing battle, without making disease the enemy, the spirits of nature have offered to bring us out of the dream of strife into the dream of wholeness" (Eliot Cowan, on the front of the pamphlet that promotes plant spirit medicine).

We checked in the dictionary and were disappointed by the definitions for the word *dream*: a distant hope or ideal, probably unattainable; a train of thoughts and fancies during sleep; to think idly. The only other word in the listed definitions that we found at all hopeful was *vision*. It helped us realise, however, just how much ground we need to cover to even remotely start reaching understanding through the medium of our industrialised language.

As people of our cultural experience it is worth our becoming aware of the crippling conditioning that separates us by even a simple word like *dream*. We are so thoroughly detached from nature, from each other, and from ourselves it's shocking. Here in the little island of Britain we are generally interested in the often changeable weather. It is an unfailing topic of conversation in any shop, pub, café, or bus stop everywhere. It's our terribly British way of belonging to place, and although it might get a bit boring, still it links us inextricably to the seasons and their energies and points to something familiar in our connection with the bigger than us world.

Robin Wall Kimmerer, Native American author of *Braiding Sweetgrass* (2015), has something to say about the language of botany, her chosen profession: "Beneath the richness of its vocabulary and its descriptive power, something is missing, the same thing that swells around you and in you when you listen to the world."

The indigenous perspective is that we are in no way separate from the dream of nature, so it's natural to listen to it. The Mbuti Pygmies who live in the Ituri rainforest of the Democratic Republic of the Congo experience their forest home as completely alive and sentient: "Moke, a wise elder, said: 'The forest is a father and mother to us, and like a father or mother it gives us everything we need—food, clothing, shelter, warmth, and affection. Normally everything goes well, because the forest is good to its children, but when things go wrong, there must be a reason'" (Colin M. Turnbull, *The Forest People*, 1961).

The coconut tree is a wonderful example of how people and nature are interlinked. Coconut is honoured wherever it grows. In the Asia-Pacific area it is known as the Tree of Life, because it provides everything people need to thrive—food, shelter, building materials and medicines. Every part of the tree has a different medicinal use. For instance, the oil is used for fever, headache, parasites, healthy bowels, skin and hair health, and cancer protection. The milk is used to treat eye infections, sore throat, and constipation. The leaves are used for muscular pain, the flowers for the kidneys, the water for bladder, immune system, and stomach as well as being great against dehydration and externally for sunburn. The roots treat gall bladder, urinary, and kidney problems, eczema, blood clots, and heartburn, and young fruits are used for stomach ache. Coconut wood is used for building. The husks are used for rope, rugs, building boards, brushes, furniture, mulch, fuel for cooking, and as a mosquito repellent. The coir, elastic fibre between the peel and the shell, can be spun into yarn and used for many things from fishing nets to car upholstery! The shells make an excellent charcoal with many uses from cooking to water filters. In every country where the coconut grows, people simply cannot comprehend how anyone could live without this tree—they are aghast to think of a country where no coconuts grow.

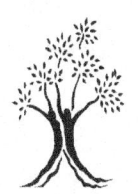

Maria helped care for my dad and his wife. She comes from the Philippines where coconuts provide for every aspect of life and she gave me a bottle of coconut oil that her sister had produced. It was like nothing I had ever used before, so rich it smelt almost like chocolate. She told me that as well as being nourishing for skin, hair, and diet and a remedy for burns, in the rainy season her mum would apply the oil to her chest and back as protection from the damp and to prevent infection. The juice of the coconut, as well as being a staple form of nourishment, is also hailed as a great hangover cure.

In our own land, the oak is one example of a mighty and versatile tree; hundreds of species of other beings live on or around an oak; the wood can be used for building homes and furniture, barrels, firewood, medicines. Acorns are a highly nutritious food: 1lb contains 2000 calories. Today, few even know that acorns are edible. In fact most of us know more about the wonders of coconut oil than we do about our own local wonder-trees. You can actually make a flour from acorns as long as you wash them first to remove the tannic acids. See Appendix B for instructions and recipe.

Watching trees through the seasons is a direct way any of us can relate to nature as the year brings its unique qualities into our daily experiences. The resonance and creative force of winter, spring, summer, harvest time, and autumn carry an energy that makes up our world as expressed through the bare branches, buds, leaves, fruits, and falling colours of our trees. These elemental forces also feature in the way our internal energy flows. Most of us know how we can feel very differently from one season to the next, the effects of changes in temperature, humidity, and light.

We are in an era of great concern about climate change and global crises connected with environmental destruction, oppressive human societies, and unprecedented extinction of our fellow species. Imbalances are writ large on the world stage just as we suffer our personal imbalances internally in our bodies, minds, and spirits. Implicit in the growing industrialisation of the last few centuries is an arrogant assumption of separation from natural law. The rising frequency of extreme climate events makes it impossible to ignore the ultimate power of nature. Opening to the deeper mysteries of the elemental forces of the seasons helps us to better connect with them and gain more understanding of our place in nature's dream, as well as learning to negotiate the inevitable losses and challenges that life brings. Working with the seasonal energies actively increases the natural flow of life, as we are no longer going against the rising and falling of the earth's cycles—even in these times of snow in May and heat wave in February. These symptomatic natural messages can be understood more as a mother's fierce guidance than a punishment from a punitive God.

One marvellous aspect of nature's power to transform is from in some cases a tiny speck of a seed to a fully rooted, stemmed, leafed, flowered, and fruited being. The blueprint encoded in the tiny seed has all it needs to manifest its life once in the favourable conditions of earth, water, air, and fire. The world is full of these multitudinous miraculous events of unceasing creativity. So too for us humans, the extraordinary miracle of procreation that results in the birth of a living, breathing human baby mirrors the natural cycles of conception, gestation, birthing, growing, maturing, ripening, withering, and dying. And as we grow we move through micro stages of these seasonal changes. As the years roll through their springs, summers, harvests, autumns, and winters, so do we. Each season brings its own flavour and qualities and these are mirrored in our lives. Behaviours and conditions that are appropriate for a toddler, for example, are not the same as for a menopausal woman; a young man emerging into adulthood needs different sorts of support and stimuli than a seven-year-old girl; an octogenarian doesn't have the same interests as an adolescent. Of course not. There is an appropriate seasonal correspondence to all development, *"To every thing there is a season, and a time to every purpose under the heaven."*

The plants know this in style. They do not need advice on how or when to bud, leaf, and flower. No one has to let them know in advance with a memo to let their leaves fall. We do not have to whisper encouragement into the winter soil in order for green shoots to appear when conditions are right. Because of these unique and unparalleled capacities is it any wonder that plants' spirits should be supremely gifted at helping us through these challenging stages at a time in human evolution when we have become very separated from nature and its dream?

The seasonal elements themselves

The Chinese five elements system grew out of a study of the way of nature. The word which has been translated as "element" really means something more like "phase" or "movement", referring to the five types of chi, life-energy, which dominate at different times. Everything in existence is made of these elements, and they cycle in an unceasing flow just as the seasons arrive, express themselves, and move on.

Each season perfectly expresses the intrinsic nature of each element. As we began to write this, midwinter approached …

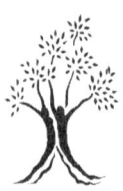

Outside it is icy cold and beginning to get dark although it is only 3 pm. The trees are bare of leaves, the landscape bleak. The energy of the earth has gone deep below. Nothing is happening on the surface. Even though the Christmas mayhem approaches, there is a pull to go quiet, to go within, to do little, to sleep more.

This is not a time for action, for doing, but for being. This is the time of water—rain washes the land clean, snow and ice freeze us into immobility. The colour is black or dark blue, the black of night. Water is life—any desert dweller knows this. The absence of water brings certain death—this can cause fear; fear has the function of keeping us alive. Water is always changing and moving—from rain to ice to snow, even from the stagnant pond it moves—evaporating into the air to come down as rain on a far-off mountain. There is a mystery to water as to life which comes, just as the spring, emerging from the earth, out of some great mystery: the source.

> *In the bleak midwinter, frosty wind made moan,*
> *earth stood hard as iron, water like a stone;*
> *snow had fallen, snow on snow, snow on snow,*
> *in the bleak midwinter, long ago.*
>
> (Christina Rossetti, 1872)

Winter walk

It's frozen down again. Just a few days ago the skies were clear with the promise of lighter, warmer days. Although still cold it felt like at least it was heading in the direction of spring; at least it might be just around the corner, as one neighbour said wistfully on passing, swaddled against the damp and chill. Snowdrops had started to go over and primrose and daffodil were emerging when suddenly down slams the freeze again. The iron cold clamps its icy grip on street and tree, on car and bush, on earth and water. This winter has been hard. It already felt relentless and now the "Beast from the East" (as people are calling this cold front from Siberia) has come calling to claim all the heat from our throats and toes, to try our hopes for reprieve and renewal that only spring can bring.

I walk out in the late afternoon, cold biting my cheeks. The air is blue, the snow-spattered hilltops blushed pink by the setting sun. The sky is clear of any cloud; there is a nearly full moon shining. Under a dusting of snow tangled webs of twigs poke out. Beneath the blanket of whiteness water is contracting into ice as I walk along the boardwalk past huge leaning willows sitting in the hardening marsh. The snow creaks and groans under the soles of my boots.

The main road momentarily cracks the spell of snow quiet with the burning roar of traffic, then it's crossed and sounds subside again, chilled silent.

Back up the hill evening approaches and the temperature drops further, contracting and stiffening movement. I feel desiccated. The orb of the moon sharpens and the white on the ground reflects upwards in the quieting light. It's bright and dark at the same time and very, very cold. Nothing stirs as night freezes itself immobile. There's a puff of smoke from a chimney, vapours from central heating outlets. Then still, quiet, shrinking as the cold intensifies. My fingers are numb in their gloves, the trees are valiant, so bare. Ice is forming underneath the snow: it's getting slippery, treacherous, harsh yet clean. It's a cold that cuts. Earlier, swirling flakes randomly filled the air dancing. Now it's sharply, seriously clear.

My dog limps on the salt-gritted tarmac: he must have a nick in his paw somewhere. Lights blink on, orange, in the town below. People are going indoors. This isn't a night to be out despite its ice-queen beauty.

The ground underfoot no longer certain, my fingers now burning with cold, I feel my legs tense against the danger of slipping as the muscles contract, no longer reliable to hold me up.

The cold has brought rigidity, no flow, still quiet on this inward and deep winter night. **Lucy Wells, 2018**

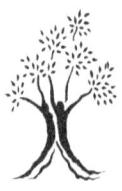

After this phase of darkness and quiet, of conserving and resting, comes the spring, the time of birth and growth. Everything erupts with green, a magnificent orchestrated medley of growth. This is the wood element—like a tree, it contains all the others within it; water is drawn up by the tree, which is made of wood. It takes the heat of the sun to make energy and it grows with its roots in the earth, from which it takes the precious minerals or metals. More than any other element, wood is the element of healing; of the growth of regeneration as well as development. Wood is upward moving, surging, vibrant. Wood is determined to grow to its full potential—and will push through any obstacles daring to impede its progress. Thus the emotion of wood is anger—the emotion arising in us when our growth is thwarted, the emotion we can use to assert our boundaries. Its colour is green.

Spring walk
As I am still unable to walk far, this "walk" comes from a series of experiences while sitting in different places in nature. I am struck by the essence I feel in each one—the bold energy, and try to convey it here. I felt it a long time ago. A pushing, pulsing urge that stirred the deep winter's waters. A big wall of energy, coming up, slowly but powerfully, infiltrating everything. Nothing escaped being enveloped by it, until finally everything and everyone was being noticeably worked by it. Faster walking, earlier rising, a well of energy inside (a feeling I must eat and drink more). On trees and bushes, buds bursting out, expressing leaves of every description. Some even flower before their leaves as a tactic to harness this precious force. Once singularly seen, birds meet in groups and chatter and sing their love and their plans for the year. They are sharp and organised as they conduct themselves. So delicate are they in a boisterous world, I can only imagine they survive by flowing with nature's forces, accurately and with no worry for yesterday or last year.

Once fully in its time, this energy commands the daily stage and fills it full of a vibrant power that is unending (it seems), showing me its truths to the exclusion of everything else, as if this is all there is. It is so easy for me to believe it. I want to. I love it—I revel in the new, powerful energy and its products—especially the masses of lush vegetation! I love to be surrounded by it, feel its bold essence, hear its buzz, sense its power—invisible yet gentle yet palpable. It expresses itself while we work, rest, and play—even while we look—and yet we don't see it growing—we are surprised by it every year, so strong and so fast! Branches and leaves reach out and touch each passer-by—"Notice me, notice me!" in a bold gesture of seeking attention. My own spirit is wooed by their vibrancy—"Join us, join us!" So I do. I'm so grateful for their power, drawing me out of the dark, slow depth of the winter's thoughtful but damp reverie.

I long to harness this precious power in a way that clears me, makes me well. After a while, just being among the throng (especially that expressed by the plants) has me feeling I am already clear and complete. I hold it in my mind and my being, giving gratitude for this gift. Everything is possible with this energy; I see only light at the end of the road (a green road at that). I'm aware of other energies and the depths I have been through, during winter, and they are past now, a distant memory, having given a basis for this forward force. Now, all I can think and be is this burgeoning power and grow in myself accordingly. Perhaps the pains I feel are resistances to this. The plants don't seem to have that issue: I observe they allow and unfold. I contemplate that, and then am whisked away into the next bold moment—there is no time to consider! Just do! OK, I get it! With regard to my own spring energy, things certainly look very different to me from this time last year (most of all, I am less fearful, and more expressive of my creativity)—so I guess my deep inner preparatory work and now going with the process could be working. **Jane Tibbotts, 2017**

I Wandered Lonely as a Cloud
I wandered lonely as a cloud
That floats on high o'er vales and hills,
When all at once I saw a crowd,
A host, of golden daffodils;
Beside the lake, beneath the trees,

Fluttering and dancing in the breeze.

Continuous as the stars that shine
And twinkle on the Milky Way,
They stretched in never-ending line
Along the margin of a bay:
Ten thousand saw I at a glance,
Tossing their heads in sprightly dance.

(William Wordsworth, 1807)

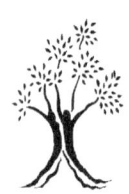

When the prolific growth of the spring, of adolescence, is over, we reach a period of maturity with the energy of summer. Everything is at its peak. Plants are in flower, attractively drawing insects and bees to them. As days lengthen and grow warmer, we come outside and are drawn to each other, to play and laugh and party. This is the energy of fire—expansive and connecting, the warmth of joy and love, fun and laughter. The red energy of the heart. As one plant spirit medicine student healer experienced:

I think it was the second or third plant that I journeyed with that I began hearing music from. I was with rosebay willowherb on a lovely sunny day. "Burn baby burn, disco inferno!" I heard as bees buzzed round. Some of them clinging to the plant, dancing in time, with their abdomens grooving back and forth. This was one groovy spirit, who appeared in very tight shiny disco trousers. Not exactly what I was expecting in the grounds of a stately home in Shropshire. **Gemma Leighton**

Poppies on the Wheat
Along Ancona's hills the shimmering heat,
A tropic tide of air with ebb and flow
Bathes all the fields of wheat until they glow
Like flashing seas of green, which toss and beat
Around the vines. The poppies lithe and fleet
Seem running, fiery torchmen, to and fro
To mark the shore.

The farmer does not know
That they are there. He walks with heavy feet,
Counting the bread and wine by autumn's gain,
But I,—I smile to think that days remain
Perhaps to me in which, though bread be sweet
No more, and red wine warm my blood in vain,
I shall be glad remembering how the fleet,
Lithe poppies ran like torchmen with the wheat.

(Helen Hunt Jackson, 1870)

Summer walk, Llanberis lake

There's a warm breeze, a blue sky, some clouds and the lake is calm. A white feather floating, purple buddleia with full conical flowers, the seed pods of sycamore, trees full of green leaves, over in the field a clump of fern, lush and green grows among pink purple thistles. I hear the sound of happy voices and traffic. Foxglove flowers hanging on, bits of litter, brambles in flower and lots of green-headed blackberries on their way as white lily-type flowers poke through the hawthorn.

The field is full of reeds and a cabbage white butterfly flutters above the pink flowers of herb robert on top of the mossy stone wall. A couple of blokes in shorts and backpacks walk their dogs past wild honeysuckle, long white and yellow petals giving off a gentle aroma. Here are yellow flowers with red spotted petals, there short purple ones with dew still on the leaves: the sun hasn't reached here yet. The cabbage white again, and a bee lands on meadowsweet. Over on a mossy tree stump brown white-edged fungi extends out from the tree. The lake is silent, birds sing, people chat, footsteps crunch on the path. Tree branches reach and dip into the water, a jogger crunches past. Moss and ivy grow on groups of trees. The gorse spines are soft. A patch of pink lilies, their flat green leaves and flowers in the process of opening, sit on an adjacent pond. Bulbous acorns are showing on oaks. For a moment there is the sense of balmy restfulness.

Torrents of ivy fall off the rock face, the holly leaves are soft. Swans are curious for food, a lady watches calmly. The sun is warm on my face; I'm glad to be out walking on this summer's day, I'm happy. Lots of people are at play on the lake, picnicking, swimming, paddling, canoeing, and noisy. A mallard and her duckling quietly paddle to the edge and cover of the plants. They stay there by the meadowsweet. Red fuschias grow wild by the roadside, some dark clouds move away across the mountains. **Emyr Roberts, PSM healer, Wales, UK**

Remember the land
Remember the land as it slept,
the wind with her rubber gloves, scrubbing,
and the trees, simplified?

The moon gained and lost,
pushed white to flow
invited young greens
for the liver's pleasure.

The orchard put on blossom,
put on its summer silver,
hid limbs so recently revealed.

The comfrey yarrow bee balm now
sing at its feet and elsewhere
vines climb crawl combine
with fern lace mugwort poison ivy.

It's all heat and multiplication
as if the ice and bone of things
were invented, an ancient myth.

Every finger of the farm
is covered in borrowed jewelry
and the eye butterflies
apple to tomato, garden to field,
unable to settle.

(Louise Berliner, 2017)

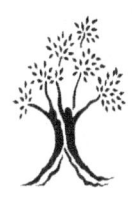

Towards the end of summer, the corn is ripening, the grass is yellowing, and the flowers have turned to fruit, an abundant harvest of maturity and ripeness. The Indian summer time of grains, berries, fruits, and nuts brings forth the bounty of the earth, which gives all nourishment and sweetness. Our Mother Earth gives us all that we need for survival; she nourishes us at her sweet breast throughout our lives. The Chinese gave the earth element the colour yellow because of the rich yellow earth of their most fertile places. We can think of the golden yellow of ripened grains rippling in our fields. Our connection to the generous outpouring the earth provides brings the security and safety of nourishment.

> *Bringing in the sheaves, bringing in the sheaves,*
> *We shall come rejoicing, bringing in the sheaves,*
> *Bringing in the sheaves, bringing in the sheaves,*
> *We shall come rejoicing, bringing in the sheaves.*

(Knowles Shaw, 1874)

An Earth walk

I wake early in the morning in my tent feeling the heavy late August dew in the dampness of my sleeping bag and the heavy stiffness in my body. Outside it is magical with a white mist rising from the distant river shrouding the valley below in mystery. The spider's webs on the brambles are jewelled with droplets. I eat my fill of the succulent berries, this is a good year for them, juicy and sweet. I compete with the spiders and flies, but there are plenty for all. The sun rises higher and burns off the river's breath so that I feel the warmth of it as the hidden valley comes into view. I love this hill near the Severn, home to many family camps every year, generously welcoming all on her lap. The hedgerow is full of activity, birds and squirrels munching and collecting. Hazel cobs are sparse this year but I make a sudden discovery of wild raspberries growing among the over-prolific Himalayan balsam. Mmmmm! My favourite. I feel full and grateful for the breakfast Mother Nature has provided. I love the Himalayan balsam actually, even though I know it's "invasive". Not only for its beautiful flowers and fragrance, but its medicine. I think of Dr Bach's reading of it, Impatiens, recommended for states of impatience, stress, and tension, when we are irritated with others and moving too quickly. It seems perfect that our fast-paced highly stressed modern world would be offered the blessing of an abundance of this remedy, relating as it does to patience and gentleness.

The sun is hot now and I find a good place to rest and feel its caress. I feel relaxed and comforted, securely held by the soft earth. I nod off to the sounds of hoverflies and bees going about their work, and the laughter of children playing in the distant camp carried to me on the warm breeze. **Pip Waller, 2012**

> *Season of mists and mellow fruitfulness,*
> *Close bosom-friend of the maturing sun;*
> *Conspiring with him how to load and bless*
> *With fruit the vines that round the thatch-eves run;*
> *To bend with apples the moss'd cottage-trees,*
> *And fill all fruit with ripeness to the core;*
> *To swell the gourd, and plump the hazel shells*
> *With a sweet kernel; to set budding more,*
> *And still more, later flowers for the bees,*
> *Until they think warm days will never cease,*
> *For summer has o'er-brimm'd their clammy cells.*
>
> (John Keats, 1819)

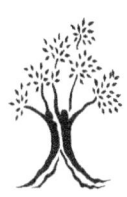

Then comes a time when the weather changes; a fresh cold sharpness is felt in the air, and we breathe deeply, feeling its purity and quality. Autumn is here, the time of winds and falling leaves, a time when all will be stripped away but the bare essentials. This is the time of metal, essence in the earth with its energy of worth and quality. The precious metals and minerals which plants drew up from the earth to grow and blossom will be returned as vegetation dies down and rots away. Metal signifies purity so has the colour white. The autumn brings the loss of leaves and light, the dying back, the onset of the dark time and is expressed as the emotion of grief, of letting go.

> *Autumn's gravity*
> *pulls down the fall*
> *til nothing remains but loss,*
> *stripped simply naked.*

An autumn walk

Sitting on a partially fallen elm trunk, being there, feeling the trees around me. It has been some time since I've been in a woodland, and I'm at home. I allow the sensations to touch me. What gifts. Rush, wind, blow it all through. Release the leaves, release the year. Chill in the air.

Colour change throughout the landscape, nature is in charge, I have no say in it. I must go with the changes, the dimming light of shorter days, the loss of playtime, the dieback of all that was blossoming and hopeful. Such harshness. I feel sad as lush growth hardens and dwindles, falling to the ground, to be met by mud and soil and mystery and eventually enveloped underground to become part of the pool of resources required for next spring's growth. As I look again, I can only admire the process.

The trees show me letting go. They are brave in their release of their leaves they have worked so hard to create. In doing so, I see they are trusting in the universe that the cycle will continue. They are part of the cycle, making it happen, and they are at the mercy of it too. They don't expect or demand, they move with the energy.

I begin to mourn the loss of all I wished to make this year, creative projects, a business, and many other things about living my life fully and truly, that didn't arise. Instead, what grew was cancer, in my breast and my bones, a shocking invasion, a distortion of health, my own system so out of balance it produced tumours in a last attempt to survive.

I mourn the loss of beautiful health and vibrancy I once had, as if all the autumn times of my life are happening in one swoop. The challenge to continue my life and regain health is huge.

I notice I'm not in sync with the woodland as I used to be; this worries and frightens me. How could I have become so disconnected?

I can do nothing but go with nature's seasonal changes, so I look again at the trees and how courageous and firm they stand. Their example gives me hope, and I choose to let go and trust in the process of life. I look again and see the opportunity this gives me to cleanse and release that which no longer serves me. This is one of many expressions of loss I need to allow. I can feel more that need to go. I must stay awake and aware to their risings and be courageous to open the door for them to leave on a vehicle called grief.

Allowing this will enable me to go into the pot of wintertime's deep meditation and sorting, and be reborn in spring in a new, healthy way. I pray I can achieve it.

I thank the trees and plants in the wood and give gratitude for my life.
Jane Tibbotts, 2016

Into the woods
Is it normal to go to the woods to cry
tears in puddles wet as the silver of a winter's sky?

grasping twigs of reassurance
which snap tender under heavy heart

falling as leaves of autumn
weep perennial grief and die again

in the sanity of seasons
where death is the smell of earth and hope the green

seeds' life becoming
all this in the woods sheltered, hidden, woven

of a thousand strands of trunk
which twinkle in the moisture of sun shards' dazzle.

Cradled in mute leaf litter
hushed by tiny creatures' sympathy, cry for a normal

which isn't anywhere to be found in handy
bite size wrappers or the concrete of a petrol station forecourt,

in all the take mistake for granted
the world's away still quietly where

the woods blossom and we stalk to talk
to tree, to earth, to sky

and know that doing this
is normal.

(Lucy Wells, 2015)

And so the wheel turns again as the water of winter returns to wash the land clean. A human being's life is also seasonal by nature: gestation in the womb mirrors the darkened internal time of winter, the force and push of birth and growth echoes the emergence of spring. Through the incredible growth of our childhood we develop to blossom into adulthood, and move out into the world to show ourselves in all our beauty and glory. Just as the warmth of summer ripens and brings forth the harvest so too are we sustained as we reap the bounty of our personal harvests and offer the fruits of our life to the world. When autumn brings the first chill and downturn, we remember the lessons of age and loss of vitality. In exchange are the wealth of experience and deeper understanding of what is essentially important as life falls back down to earth and we prepare to encounter the final loss of our life itself as winter.

Or at least that is how it potentially can flow. Which one of us could say we have had a smooth and natural transition of these phases in our lifetime experience? Just as we see weather patterns change and deregulate so it seems we are now so often lost in these cycles in our own lives.

The offering of the plant spirits is to bring the gifts of the seasons into the rhythm of our lives, just as nature dreams it, helping us in turn release from some of our human nightmares.

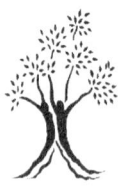

Season Song

I

*When you wake in springtime to the singing of the birds
And the wind is in the trees and voices can be heard,
If you listen closely, there are voices all around—
Voices flying through the air and rising from the ground.*

*The world's alive, the world's alive,
You hear those voices say.
Come in to life, come in to life,
Come in to life today.*

*When you hear those voices, there's one thing you can do—
Open up your heart to life and let life open you.*

II

When you're in the garden and the summer sun is high
And you're working hard and the sweat gets in your eyes,
Through the sweat you see that life is growing all around—
Flower and fruit and seed and root are growing from the ground

The world is growth, the world is growth,
It's growing every way.
Grow into life, grow into life,
Grow into life today.

When you see that growing, there's one thing you can do—
Open up your heart to life and let life grow in you.

III

In the autumn evening when you're sitting by the fire
And the leaves are on the ground and chill is in the air,
Everything is changing as the wood's transformed by flame—
Heat and light and smoke and ash, nothing can stay the same.

The world is change, the world is change,
It's changing every way.
Transform your life, transform your life,
Transform your life today.

When you feel that changing, there is one thing you can do—
Open up your heart to life and let life transform you.

IV

In the winter midnight when you're warm inside your bed
And the ground is cold outside and everything looks dead,
As you drift you start to dream the world is dreaming too
And in that dream the dreaming world is dreaming life anew.

The world's a dream, the world's a dream,
It's dreaming through the dark.

*Dream into life, dream into life,
That is your sacred work.*

*When you dream that dreaming there is one thing you can do—
Open up your heart to life and let life dream through you.*
(Jonathan Merritt, 2017–18)

We invite you to connect with the energy of the current season.

Make space of at least an hour to walk, sit, swim, cycle, outside in as natural an environment as is possible for you. Notice the smells, the colours, the sounds, the feelings that arise in you in response to this particular time of year. Come home and represent this in some creative way. Write, draw, photograph, sing, a description of your observations. Even if you haven't done anything arty since junior school, have a go. This kind of expression can bypass the busy mind and allow the felt sense of heart experience to come through. Try not to judge your creations, celebrate them as you would a young child's offerings. Repeat this exercise in every season—spring, summer, late summer or harvest time, autumn, and winter.

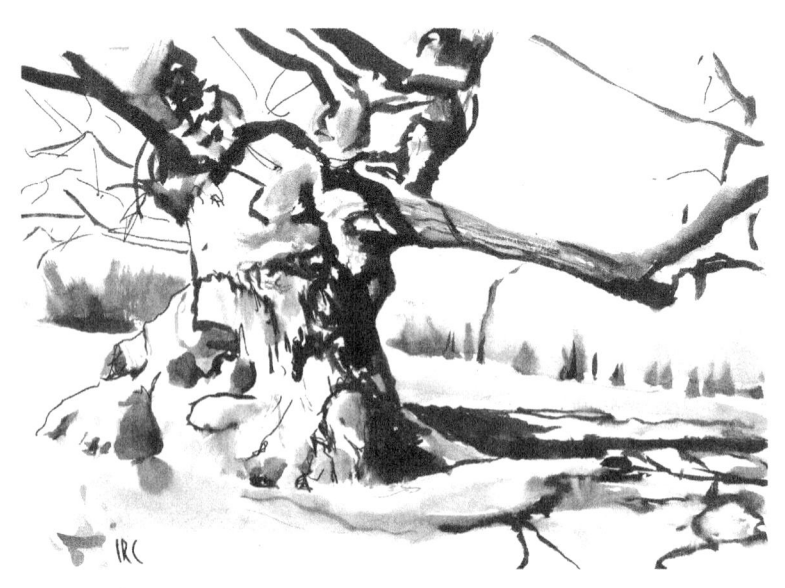

Winter Tree by Ian Collett.

CHAPTER FIVE

Meeting the plant spirits—the shamanic dream journey

The juice of PSM comes from the healers' friendship with the plants themselves. It is understood by indigenous healers that this relationship is key; plant medicine won't work without it. Eliot Cowan tells a story about American adventurer Peter Gorman, on a wild-boar hunt in the Amazon. While they were out the Matses Indian he was with pointed out dozens of plants he used for medicines. Back in the village Peter gets his notebook and asks the Amazonian shaman to repeat the information so he could learn from it. Eliot continues:

> The hunter-shaman smiles at Peter and then begins to laugh. He invites all his wives and children over to have a good laugh, too. When they have all laughed themselves out, he explains, "That was just to introduce you to some of the plants. If you want to actually use a plant yourself, the spirit of the plant must come to you in your dreams. If the spirit of the plant tells you how to prepare it and what it will cure, you can use it. Otherwise, it won't work for you. That was a good one! I've got to remember what you just said!" He laughs again. (Eliot Cowan, *Plant Spirit Medicine*, 2014)

Plants as we see, smell, feel, taste, and know them in the material world of our everyday life have souls, spirits, energies, that go far beyond what our ordinary senses can engage with. This is knowledge that indigenous people know in the same way that we know how to read and write and cross the road safely. In the words of Canadian herbalist Michael Vertolli, who works in a way very close to indigenous herbal tradition:

> Let's just say that all of the plant medicines that I work with reveal themselves as distinct beings—even the ones that I don't work with but am in relationship with every day because they live on the land. They are all part of the medicine because they are part of the land that the medicine comes from. There are also other chief spirit helpers that are not plants. They are animals, sacred sites and ancestral spirits of the land.

We have a way to meet the plant spirits and build such friendships. As trainee plant spirit medicine healers we learn an elemental language they understand in order to discover their medicine. We learn this within a rigorous diagnostic protocol that leads us to better relate to the needs of our patients. Whilst this is complicated, the building of relationship with plants is a wonderful pastime which anyone can do to enrich their connectedness with the natural world.

It is begun by what we call a "plant study". This is a development of the earlier exercises found on p. 7 and 39. The full plant study includes time spent outdoors with a plant, ideally in its wild growing state. Utilising all the senses we pay very close attention to everything about the plant. This type of observation was pioneered by the philosopher poet and playwright Goethe in the nineteenth century.

> We must first encounter the plant and thoroughly describe its physical manifestation in fine detail as it appears to our senses. This is a process of painting the plant into our mind, so that we know the outer shapes, colours and textures of the root, shoot, leaf, flower and fruit. This mode of observation is similar to the methods of the artist, who is able to see, and therefore paint, with such insight into the whole ... Through the practice of visualising the plant in our mind's eye, we can actively melt the boundaries between each part and experience the plant in the whole of its developmental processes; the plant growing through time ... Thus we move from perceiving the plant directly with our senses as a solid, separate

object, to exploring the mysterious fluid realm of its metamorphosis through time as it grows within us. This experience is often accompanied by a strong physical sense of the plant-being growing within you ... (Natasha Myers, *Exploring Goethean Science*).

Having announced your intention to the plant spirits, go on your walk until you feel called by a particular plant. The call can come in many ways, often something as simple as being particularly attracted to it. Introduce yourself out loud with your name, and make an offering to the plant in anticipation of the exchange which will take place—you're not just taking something for nothing. The traditional offering to plant spirits in Britain is some barley or oat seeds. In the Americas it is tobacco. Identify the plant if you can and begin to observe it closely; notice how the plant is growing, who are its neighbours; draw and paint it; smell, feel, taste (if you know it's edible). Make sure to ask permission to pick some—even if you feel silly doing this. Just ask the question and allow an answer to come to you. Respect if you get a no. Pay attention to every detail—the weather, anyone who turns up, anything that happens in the course of your experience. Relax and do what you can to merge with the plant, daydream a little with it—the aim is to enter the dream of the plant itself. Afterwards write down every part of your experience.

It is a warm sunny day in May and the nettles here are strong and vigorous. I'm remembering all the meals these plants have given me and my family this year, nourishing and uplifting. The smell, as I rub the leaves, is sweetly scorched and I roll the leaf between my fingers to remove the sting and have a chew, I find the taste to be sweet, broad, and earthy-green. After a while I feel gentle heat in my throat. My fingers tingle with the sting, an aliveness and zing, warming. I see that they grow in big communities in edge places, enjoying a mixture of sun and shade; they spread like wildfire. They stand so straight. Clivers, the sticky weed grows here, they often grow together I have noticed. I can see lots of little holes and nibble marks on the leaves, they have been munched by insects, who I wonder? I know that they are a favourite food of many caterpillars. They need to have the sting for their own protection but I guess they protect others too who live on them. I feel their generosity to humans and that, like fire, they can bite with their sting if they are not respected. As I sit with the nettles here I feel gratitude and friendship. I feel them to be both in and around me in protective companionship. They have strong spirit and stand upright and purposeful.

As I introduced myself to this tiny blue flower with a white centre, I was overcome with a feeling of peacefulness and stillness. The plant began to open up to me and informed me that it closed itself on rainy days and opened to the sunlight. I felt its quiet assurance, telling me everything was going to be just fine. And yet, it also said it was a little scared, revealing the flip side of its calmness. Considered a weed by many, and so small that most people step right over it without even knowing it is there, it was a well and wealth of knowledge and depth. "I can cry easily, I get so scared. I am beauty, I am peace, I am depth. I fall deep in love, to the reservoirs of peace. I bring calm and relaxation to those who are anxious and movement and fear to those who need that. Sometimes I don't know what I have to offer, that is why I am so scared. I bend but can easily be crushed. I protect myself. I am Speedy Gonzales. I come quickly and fold up just as quickly. One minute I'm there and one minute I'm not. I race here, I race there." Not yet knowing what to make of those words, I continued to lie there, staring at the clouds, daydreaming. My mind floated, my focus drifted. I could no longer retain what was being said, I was just being in a very, very relaxed state. When I came to, I felt deeply refreshed.

A squeaking stops me. I have been walking quite quickly up the beautiful wooded valley, stepping from rock to rock and dodging fallen trees as I climb upwards on the soft mossy path. I am still now, taking in the chill, the damp atmosphere, and lush green plants by the fast running stream. But who is it that is speaking? Two tall oaks rubbing bodies, their voices persistent and urgent call me. Slender trunks, reaching to sunlight, silhouetted, dark and determined, softly cloaked in ivy and moss. They wave in a hypnotic, slow, gentle rhythm as the wind catches their branches, stilling my mind and opening my senses. I hear the rushing burble of the stream and the ever changing breath of the wind. I see clouds dance through the clear blue sky. I feel the breeze gently licking my body and cooling the skin on my face. Birds caw and twitter, my breath rises then falls as it enters and leaves my body. Feet firmly on the ground I find myself responding to the waving trees. As I sway back and forth the wind blows stronger as if to say "Hello" as it often does when I honour its presence. I am dropping into the dream of nature. My heart softens and expands; I become increasingly aware of being part of this. I am the trees, I am the stream, I am the river, I am the earth, and I am also myself. I am aware of the familiar feeling of subtle, blissful, light energy that comes when I give a plant spirit medicine treatment.

We were training and we had to go to this plant, a very prickly plant. I'd forgotten to ask it if I could pick some. I'd forgotten to ask it. And this plant just said, "Grrrr! Bugger off!" and I thought, "Wow! It spoke to me. It really spoke to me." I hadn't done the protocol. So I said, "I'm really sorry, can we try again." And then it was OK for me to continue. That is the first time a plant actually spoke to me, and it was very angry that I'd picked it without asking, without taking care.

The experience of being with the plant as it grows is followed up by a shamanic dream journey with a drum, using the Michael Harner method. Journeying is a simple tool most people can learn as a way to deepen connection with what Harner termed "non-ordinary reality", and which most indigenous people call "the spirit world". Some people are able to "journey" immediately while others find they need a lot of practice and experience unsuccessful attempts before being able to enter the dream world. Relaxed perseverance is the key to success. Harner found on studying shamanic methods from indigenous people in many parts of the world that a common tool for entering non-ordinary reality involved use of a drum beat at a particular frequency. It turns out that when we listen to a rhythm of 120–240 beats per minute, our brainwaves change to the theta waves of a trance state—what Harner calls a shamanic state of consciousness.

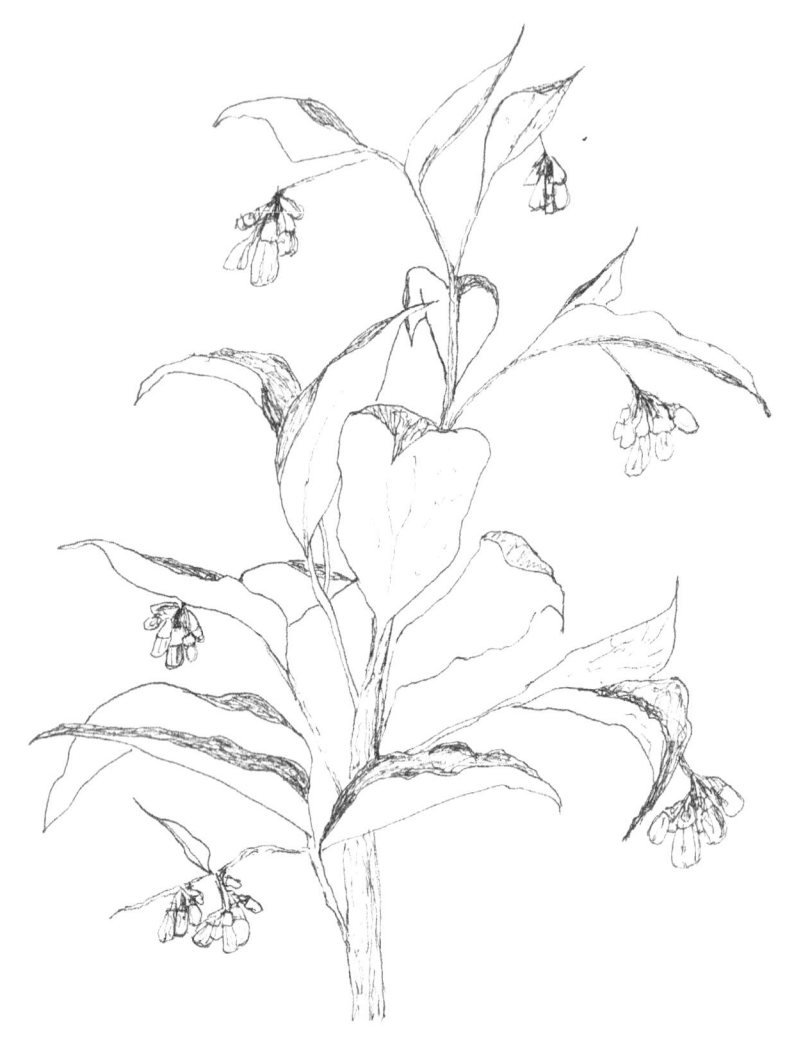

Comfrey by Michael Locke.

Some people find it easy to trust their experience, some see things very vividly, for others the sensations are more subtle and may be vaguer. Many may find it more complicated to get into a zone where the mind isn't dominating with its busy blah blah blah trying to persuade that we are simply "making it up". People journey in different ways, feeling, thinking, seeing, or hearing and it's important to simply give yourself over to the dream with a childlike openness, allowing

Do this indoors or somewhere you won't be interrupted. You either need your own drum (and drummer if possible) to beat a repetitive rhythm, or you can listen to a recording. For some, ten minutes is an ideal length for this kind of journey, others may need longer. It is customary for the journey to end with a signal known as the call-back, followed by some very rapid drumming for about a minute as you return to ordinary reality. (Michael Harner's book, The Way of the Shaman, *1992).*

This method allows us to enter the dream of the plant still further and build a relationship with it as a spirit ally. State your intention—"to journey to meet with the spirit of the plant" you just spent time with. You might do this out loud and repeat it three times to anchor it clearly in your mind. Start the drumming, sit or lie comfortably and begin by imagining yourself to be standing in a place you know that reminds you of the earth. Look around for some kind of opening into the ground—it might be a rabbit hole or other entrance to an animal burrow, a cave, a hollow tree, a pool of water you could dive into. Entering through the opening you find yourself in a tunnel—go down the tunnel and for whatever might happen to be received and noted.

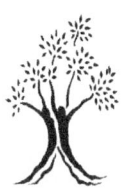

I had seen a plant that I thought I'd work with but someone got to it before me. I knew I was running out of time to do the study so I saw a small clump of speedwell and as I sat down next to it I mentally said to myself, "Oh well, you'll have to do." I picked a small piece to journey with when the study was over. This was my first journey to the plant spirits and I found myself being pulled straight through the earth until I came out into a wooded landscape with dappled sunlight. I seem to be in a lane. I watch as the most beautiful ethereal woman with long black hair, alabaster skin, and long blue and white flowing gown approached me. I asked her if she was the spirit of the speedwell and she replied she was. I asked her if she had a message for me and she said, "There is beauty in even the smallest of things." Once we had returned from the journey I left the room in tears, because I realised that I had had a most gentle rebuke and a reminder not to overlook how beautiful even the smallest thing can be and it does not always have to be big and bold to be beautiful.

keep on until you come out into a landscape. This is the landscape of what Harner termed the lower world. Pay attention to the sights, sounds, and smells, and begin to look around you. If you get distracted and forget what you are doing, repeat your intention.

Somewhere near the growing plant you will find its spirit. Introduce yourself and spend some time getting to know it. Often in journeys we are shown things rather than told. Information or guidance that comes in dream journeys can be very explicit but is commonly symbolic and takes practice to interpret and understand. Do what you can to resist all temptation to think about what's happening until later. When the call-back comes, swiftly return the same way you went until you feel you are fully back in your body, then write down every detail. Afterwards you can ponder the meanings revealed to you—but it's not necessary to do this in order to benefit.

I went to meet hawthorn. I decided to climb as high as I possibly could and then some more. The hawthorn trees were calling me, "Not this one, not this one, up and up—there!" I climbed as high as I could and it was there! She was in blossom, it was heady, the scent. Like hah! Gorgeous. I turned round and there was just the most magnificent view. My time there was great. Then I journeyed: I was looking up, and there was a waterfall coming down, there was a stillness to this waterfall, it was water and it was fire, it was hot, like Mexico. I climbed up this hill, and there was a beautiful maiden. A woman like Mother Mary, a figure that walked through the crevice of where one boulder met another; there was slate everywhere. At the very top I could see a dark cathedral like a Buddhist temple structure. I reached another plateau and then suddenly this boulder turned into a gorilla! It had such peace about it, completely and utterly happy to be who and where he was. He looked at me, completely content. I went towards him and to another area, looking out on a plain, still this feeling of peace. I came out of the journey feeling really peaceful, I was really moved, and wrote it down. Then I looked at the picture that I'd drawn up on the hill in "real" waking life, and lo and behold that maiden was in the drawing and I hadn't even realised. I didn't draw the maiden, but when I looked at it there she was.

My wife took me to a herb day at a local community garden. We were making elderberry rob and hawthorn ketchup in this lovely valley. It was a wonderful experience. Towards the end of the day we were taken on a journey to a hawthorn tree, and taught how to connect with this tree, to do a shamanic journey. It was my first one. I was soon into the dreamtime, went down a rabbit hole under the ground. I got to a wooden door and went through it, and there was a man standing there. A little man with a long nose, lumps and bumps and slightly overweight, and there was a table. I knew what to do, so I lay on the table and he started covering me with this gloop, mashed up hawthorn berries. He was covering me all over and I just lay there in this little warren and let this little man cover me in these berries, and it was wonderful. That was my first experience of having a shamanic journey and I found it easy, it just happened—this guy turned up and it was beautiful and he was just happy to give me healing.

My relationship to the world is in general very kinaesthetic. When I do a journey to a plant I often feel a lot of sensation in my body. One example of this is in relation to a fire plant that I work with. In my dream journey, I experienced a lot of joy and pleasure. The plant spirit anointed and massaged my body, followed by a swim in a bubbling jacuzzi-like part of the river.

I always loved plants. Journeying was very easy. Overall I felt like I was meeting friends. Each of them was so different. There were times I felt like I'd met something so pure and so good and so intelligent that it infused my body. Every time I went out to study with a plant I felt I was given something. It felt all of them were a different aspect of me, of life.

Once you get the hang of it journeying is a rich and rewarding spiritual activity. The following stories give a taste of the variety and beauty of the sorts of experiences people encounter when connecting with plants in this way. We are naming the plants but not the human storytellers to give the plants centre stage. The journeys reflect the astonishing variety of plant forms on our planet, and our individual ways of relating with them, and some tell of unusual places where non-ordinary and ordinary realities overlap.

Wild cherry Coming out into an area with hundreds of enormous cherry trees, I see the most beautiful white flowers. I suddenly realise that I am slowly rising on one of these flowers. I seem to be inside one of the trees and I'm rising at a much faster rate. I get the impression that I'm in an elevator and there are watery windows in the tree shining with translucency so it looks like there is nothing there. I see green all around me. I travel higher and higher until the elevator stops and I can see an old man with white robes and a long white beard. He is holding a white gnarly staff in his right hand. I mentally ask him if he is my spirit guide. He points outward with his staff indicating that I should look and I cannot believe that the world is so full of plants and flowers; the view is breathtaking and I feel so small, as if any impact I could make would not even cause a ripple. Suddenly I'm moving again, I'm being shown landscape after landscape and coastline with green everywhere I look. I have no idea where any of these places are but I get a feeling for the vastness of the land. As soon as I have this realisation I find myself falling and I drop into the ocean. I'm not worried about being under the water, I can still breathe. I look around and see buildings like skyscrapers and smaller ones, decaying and crumbling; there is life growing on these buildings. I feel myself start to rise until I am once again back on land where there are more derelict buildings. I notice that the plants are actually growing and spreading over the buildings as if claiming back the land. To my right is a small beach area. Suddenly a huge whale beaches itself in front of me and for the longest time I'm held by the gaze of its one eye. After a while the whale back flips into the sea and is gone. Suddenly I seem to be travelling up again on the cherry flower, higher and higher until eventually I look down and can see chinks of golden bright light emanating from the planet. The light starts in chinks and cracks at first and then it slowly spreads, merging to turn into one bright ball of light whose luminosity reaches ever upwards towards the sun.

Welsh poppy As I sat with the poppy I first felt hugely tired and fell asleep. I felt a deep wound, a terrible grief, then I was restless. I daydreamed and saw the land soaked with blood, a warrior of light standing in a field of blood, dead children and babies all around. Very disturbing. Later in the journey I come out in a dry and barren landscape, different to other journeys, I usually come out into a clearing in a forest. It's a wasteland. Long years, centuries, millennia of battles. A deep weariness comes on me, having to move on again. The poppy spirit appears as a Celtic warrior. He is sitting, slumped over, defeated, but somehow I also see him standing straight and tall. So many ravaged peoples and lands. Deeply sad. The horror and futility of war. Blood stains the ground. He said, there's a need to stop promoting war on any side. Don't take sides, it just adds to the polarisation. Even being anti-war is taking a position somehow. There's no sides. Taking sides keeps conflict going. I heard in my head a song that I learned thirty years ago from my herbalist friend Calder Bendle: "I've never been anywhere, I've never done anything. Cried too few tears, smiled too few smiles, in this place for two thousand years." Then the call-back came. I said goodbye to the Welsh poppy warrior and thanked him.

Red clover I feel myself going down a long narrow, deep burrow. It's full of roots and I see earthworms moving by me. It's hot and cramped and suddenly I fall into a more open space of purple/pink cushions creating an inviting place to rest. I ask if I can rest here because I feel so tired and a voice answers me. I can't see where it's coming from at first, then I see a hedgehog close by. Its prickles are purple and pink. They are the petals of the clover flowers. It was sweetly scented and as I looked it spread its front paws to open wide and stretch around me in a shield like, protective cloak. He enveloped me into the cloak and I was inside the hedgehog. I became the hedgehog and out into a meadow. The flowers were all around me, above me as I crawled through the meadow surrounded by my friends. I was not alone. The plants were all talking to me and I felt safe amid them in my hedgehog protective armour. I would be protected and safe and rested with my prickle armour and I could always call on it, red clover, hedgehog heart protector, for my kindness towards hedgehogs in my own garden. The drum quickened and I came back into the room. Later that night when I went to get into my car I heard a rustling noise nearby and saw that there was a large shape in the way. I thought it was a rock but knew I wasn't to stand on it. As I opened the car door the light illuminated the shape. A huge hedgehog sat in my path, unmoving despite the noise and light. I bent down to talk to it and thank it for my protection earlier and gently moved it away from the path of my wheels and drove home smiling and happy.

Sweet violet As I lay down with these lovely violets in the sunshine I felt, or saw, a haze of purple violet colour, I felt sweet and mellow. I could hear jazz saxophone music wafting from somewhere nearby, it seemed the perfect fit for it. What a lovely flower, sweet and delicious and loving. Simple pleasures and easiness. I went into a daydream and felt myself with a tiny violet fairy, so friendly and welcoming. She gave me a drink of violet. I never tasted anything so deliciously lovely. A wave of deep sadness came over me as I thought of how few violets there are in our world now and felt the lack of opportunity to be with them. I cried and felt something about being able to really let myself know deeply that I truly have people in my life. I felt some people who are close to me, felt how I can't let their love in, can't feel it coming in. I felt the heartbreak of letting go of an old lover, the bitterness, then a releasing of a feeling of trying to "get" something that was just not available. Later in the journey, I went into a very dark, green, still, ancient woodland and came to a huge bank of violets growing among moss beneath a canopy of oak trees. The violet spirit appeared as a very warm and loving woman wearing purple. I began to cry; she encouraged me to keep crying. "Just keep crying, there's no shame you need to feel about being heartbroken." I cried about every heartbreak of my life. I felt stuck in heartbreak and loss. Every time I stopped myself crying, she encouraged me to continue by her sheer kindness. My tears formed a huge pond. I asked her,

"What can I give you?" She said, "You are giving me your tears, such richness!" The pond became a lake, a glistening beautiful lake of jewels, a fairy wonderland. All the tears of heartbreak filled the lake with the treasures of those lost and broken dreams, making the lake beautiful. I felt a softening and an acceptance of feeling heartbroken, that it's OK to feel this sadness, there is a beauty in it. I felt a simple pleasure at being alive.

Motherwort When I went to the lower world and I called out to motherwort, she came towards me through a motherwort plant as tall as her. Many spirits encircled me all white and shimmery. They touched me and I became like them. I asked mother what her medicine is and she points to my heart and says "I fix problems with heart—sadness, grief, etc., any problems." She kept stroking me, loving me. She lay me down, I was obviously a child. She wanted me to just relax and let her love me but I couldn't do it, I felt uncomfortable. I couldn't take in the love she was trying to give me. I was having trouble keeping my identity, I couldn't keep my vision of who or where I was. She told me that I should take in the love that she was giving me because I was safe and secure. She was so gentle and accepting, loving me totally unconditionally, I wanted to be able to take it in. She smiled all the time with this beautiful radiant smile. She had perfect white teeth. However, I never felt safe or secure, I couldn't relax, I felt edgy and nervous. I couldn't just be, I couldn't accept her loving and caring.

Nettle As I follow the drumbeat and relax I travel downwards in the dark earth and come out in a warm sunny garden. I'm drawn along a pathway and meet a little grandmother with white hair, a shawl, and big skirts; her eyes twinkle with friendliness and humorous mischief. She asks me to follow her and we climb a ladder propped against her cottage wall. She is fast and energetic. Then there is another ladder and another ladder. We are climbing high into the sky. She eventually stops and asks me what I see. We look down and can see the land far below us. I have a moment of lurching fear. "Ask your heart," she says. I look down again and see that the green land is shaped like an enormous hand. "What else do you see? Ask your heart." ... I relax, I see clearly that the earth is the mother who holds us all and is the connection between all beings here. "Now", she says, "jump!" I jump and my feet immediately hit the ground. She is laughing and laughing, "Everything is not what it seems." I am filled with a true belly laugh. I laugh out loud and joy runs through my body. She tells me how she and the many plant spirits are connecting the land together and that she can help people who feel far away and removed. She offers connection. She is a highly protective and loving spirit. She is full of warmth and joy. Before I leave I ask if there is anything I can do for her and she asks me to tell people about her.

Ash tree I have a large garden populated with many native trees including ash. I was naturally drawn to the hawthorn and the elder, I quite liked the hazel, but felt the ash was a bit pushy and not my "kind of tree"! My first real communication with a plant spirit was in Glastonbury when I spent a day with Eliot. The plant Eliot took us to work with was an ash. We did a daydream first beside the tree. I felt ash had a central "core of knowing" and I had a sense of energy moving up and down from Earth Mother through the roots, the trunk, connecting to Sky Father. I loved the dappled sunlight sparkling through the leafy leaflets, creating diamonds and an airy space right down to the ground. It felt as if there were layers of light, wisdom, and truth. And then I met the spirit of this tree. He was a little elderly man with spectacles on the end of his nose, a round tummy, and a big round face that reminded me of the world, friendly, full of sparkling energy, sitting with one leg crossed over the other and looking at me quizzically, raising an eyebrow and winking at me, "Oh, is that so? So you really think that's it do you? Ha ha, really?" Laughing and jolly, he told me to look through the layers, for the core of the matter, what's really going on, what's the truth here? Question more to find the truth. Back inside for the drumming journey later, I journeyed down and came out in a glade of ash trees, introduced myself, and apologised for not making the time to say hello to the ash trees in my own garden ... and that little man appeared sitting at the foot of the oldest tree and said "Oh, I know!" We flew up above the earth and he showed me blackened areas, the polluted earth, sea, smoke in the skies—dark patches among the blue and green, then we flew over the Amazon and the trees were crying—I felt so sad but what could I do? "Don't accept things at face value, always question, dig deeper for the truth, talk to and challenge people about their actions, in a positive way, and sow seeds to germinate and grow, seeds of truth, knowledge for the planet, sow seeds for the children, to grow within them. Use me to help people find their truth, I'll support them and heal them as they go through the pain of knowing." Ash then went and sat under his tree and smoked a long pipe. Eliot told us later that Ash is the holder of ancestral wisdom, about connectedness, how to live without separateness which leads to misguided human actions.

Yew I noticed that the yew trees were in flower and I decided I would do a plant study. I found a yew tree that was over 1,000 years old, in the graveyard of an old church in a rural Shropshire village. It was impressively beautiful and ancient. They are called the trees of eternity as they form a ring with time, a ring of yew, with a hollow centre. Because of this, yew trees are associated with immortality, and everlasting life. I sat in the sun and drew the yew. I gave thanks to it, felt it, sat with it. I did not taste it as yews are poisonous. When I was ready I climbed inside and lay down within its gnarled and wondrous inside, completely obscured and hidden from the outside world. It felt amazing to be curled up within this ancient being. Maybe because of this my journey was quick and very clear. I climbed inside a big grave, and walked down a spiral staircase, down, down to the underworld. I enter into the black, and emerge flying, I am a raven. I soar around the skies, feeling the joy of flight, and then land in my nest that is made within the branches of the yew tree.

The yew spirit appears, much like the images of the green man. He has a tree form, but a kind bearded face with twinkling eyes. We are friends and it feels good to be with him and to swing in his moving branches. I ask him what his medicine is that he can offer me in my healings. "Fly little one," he said. "Go see what you can find!" And so I flew off and came to a city, an ancient city. In every house that I looked into I saw people who were sad and crying, who were depressed and miserable. It was as though there was no light in anybody's heart. I flew back to the yew, and he came with me to the city, and breathed over the people. The light returned in their eyes, they became happy again. They stopped crying and being sad; purpose returned.

He said to me, "I give you the power to see what needs to change and the capacity to change it. Vision and change." I thanked him. He gave me a yew berry as a gift, and I flew with it in my raven beak, back into the darkness, where I changed back to a human. Climbing the spiral staircase, I return back into the world, back into the soft gnarled underbelly of the ancient yew. Gratitude fills my heart.

The above are examples of using the plant study and dream journey to connect with and experience the plants very directly. The following stories reveal how the dream of nature enters our reality, both from our active communication and without any deliberate decision such as in daily happenings or in our night-time dreams.

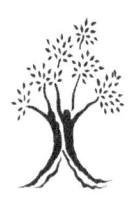

It was early summer. I had been taught how to study and journey with the plants and this was the season to do it, so I was out and about on a regular basis, to wander childlike in nature looking for plant friends to make the acquaintance of. As can happen with regularity, a sense of habit had set in which can dull the magic. It's so easy to tarnish. And so this day I found myself putting off departure from the house in favour of busying myself with little jobs. So easily done, there's always washing up or clothes to hang out, quick phone calls or texts to send. I had a deadline to collect my young son from school and I started to push against the clock, a familiar habit. I was so often compromising myself with unnecessary duress with this stressful methodology. By the time I had got out of the house I hardly had enough time to find, connect, draw, study, be with the plant, let alone return home and journey with the drum. Nevertheless, out there on the hill I found an enchanting clump of sweet violets basking in a sunny spot and sat down to begin. But my mind was ticking away, ever on the clock. I drew and looked at this pretty plant with half my attention on getting to the school on time, just like chatting to someone but looking over their shoulder expecting to see something else. I was just coming down off the hill, reckoning on my timing being about right for the school run, when I saw an elderly gentleman about to embark on the steep uphill stretch. He was walking laboriously slowly. Not someone I recognised, in itself unusual as I knew most of the old folk in my small town by sight at least. His white shirt was open at the collar and although clearly quite frail he had no walking stick. What struck me as I drew up close to him was the vibrant deep violet colour of his eyes and the sense of sharp relief around his outline that made him stand out from the trees and hill of the background. "Good afternoon," he said excruciatingly slowly. "I've just been in hospital." There was a twinkle in his brilliant eyes. "I've decided to come out for a little constitutional, to build myself up again." "Ah, good for you," I said hurriedly, hoping to put a stop to any further chat and get away quickly, but before I could stroll off with anything even slightly resembling kindly politeness he was replying, "It was open heart surgery they did …" and launched into a painstaking description of his illness and the whole story. Each word seemed an eternity as my insides strained to hurry away and get on with what I was doing, quickly, to get it done … At some point in the encounter, however, I felt a surrender inside me: he was a very engaging personality and what after all was a few minutes to spare an elderly person with such pluck and courage? The hurrying vibe dissipated and I figured the plant study didn't matter as much as caring to listen. It was then that he let go of my attention. "Well, I mustn't keep you," he smiled knowingly, his eyes shining, and started off towards the steep slope. I walked off feeling strangely altered and didn't look back because I knew that he wouldn't be there. I returned home with plenty of time to write up my experience and get to school with a deep sense of peace and spaciousness inside.

Nettle is the first wild plant I connected with in my late teens when I set out on the road. I discovered deep love for the wild plants and passion to learn how people used them in the past for food and medicine. I devoured the field guides and books I could find about their uses and soon discovered nettles, which I obsessively gathered and made into soup for all my friends, wading into their midst and even enjoying the tingle of their sting. I loved them. Many years later, Eliot's book found its mysterious way into my hands and it was not long before he became my teacher. Eliot taught us how to journey to the spirit of the plants and then we embarked on our own adventures to befriend our local plants. I set out to the nettle patch at the wild end of my garden and did a plant study and journey. Some months later the nettle came and showed me things in my dreams during the deep part of the night. In the dream I have two nettle stems in my hands, one from a male plant and one from the female. They can be used to help bring balance between the male and female within a person when they have become confused. Next I am being taken by the nettle spirit through the sky in an intense windy storm. There are blossom petals flying about as I fly over trees. I'm taken to see Eliot and told I must tell him about an experience I had with a storm when I was eighteen. After this the nettle takes me onwards to see a friend in need and how to help her. She shows me how she is a protective spirit. On the strength of this dream I was prompted to talk to Eliot who sent me for a divination which led to the beginning of another unfolding chapter of connection with the weather, but that is another story. What is still astonishing to this day is how the nettle knew about my path and helped me to find my way.

Daisy was one of the first herbs that I really noticed talking. We were out in a beautiful daisy meadow. So many daisies you wouldn't believe. We hadn't heard anything about daisy being used for medicine but we thought we'd harvest some and see what we felt. They were enchanting, making these delicious "pop, pop, pop" sounds as we popped off their heads. We collected them into our baskets and it was like we couldn't stop. There was something compulsive about it—we filled these baskets. We had to leave, but we ended up late because we couldn't stop—we kept going back for just another handful. There were still thousands of daisies left; it felt like we'd hardly touched the sides of the meadow, that's how many there were. But there was something in it, like those compulsive behaviours where you're aware of them but you just can't stop. So we looked at Dr Edward Bach's work and sure enough there under bellis perennis, the common daisy, he said daisy helps to release repeated patterns of behaviour.

After my daughter's passing I started studies of herbalism and working as a volunteer in a hospice. I found that when I would just be doing reiki, or sitting in silent prayer with someone who was dying, sometimes a plant would show up. It was really quite beautiful. I would later ask the person if that meant anything to them. Every time without fail they had a deep relationship with that tree or that particular plant in their garden, perhaps a garden they'd had years before, or they grew up with. For instance with one particular person this mighty oak tree came in and I told her about it and she said, "I used to go and sit in the base of that tree when I was a kid, and it was where I would hide and be held, and it just protected me." And she said that she hadn't thought about it in a long time, and it was really beautiful to see the plant come for her.

My mother died of cancer in a Dorothy House hospice. The first night after dying she was put into a "freezer" room to rest before being moved to the morgue. I took a vase of closed freesias into the room. I wanted her to have them with her as they were one of her favourite flowers, even though I thought they were likely to die in the cold. Next morning I went in to see her and the moment I opened the door I was assailed by an overpowering scent of freesia. Every flower had opened, something I have never seen before or since. I felt very strongly that this was a communication from her to me through the plant world.

I was sitting with my back against a tree on Hampstead Heath. I had been focusing on my breathing, my spine, and the contact of my back with the tree and had been there for about an hour or so when I became aware that I had moved into a different state. I distinctly heard the tree suggest I get up and go to one of its neighbours several hundred metres away. As I moved to follow this I saw out of the corner of my vision a man, there were several people passing but he was the one my brain noted. I went to the recommended tree quickly, was about to sit when this one suggested I keep moving to another one. As I moved I saw the same character approaching. This happened with several other trees by which time it was clear he was pursuing me. The trees were guiding me off the Heath. Just as I was reaching an exit the man came hurriedly out of some bushes with his trousers down.

Here in Seattle the winters are very cool and rainy, but the summers are dry and hot, and like a Garden of Eden. Flowers pop up out of the sidewalk. Trees bear fruit along the city streets. Among gardeners and plant enthusiasts, along with the beauty and lush growth of the summer, comes a slew of "invasive" species, non-native plants that have found the cool winters and hot summers irresistible. One of these is the Himalayan blackberry, a spiny thicket that through the smallest amount of wrangling gashes the hands and arms; and it can grow roots from the tiniest cutting, so eradication is nearly impossible. One particularly warm summer, it started growing up against the side of our house, high up and nearly covering the whole side of our roof. As a PSM healer, I of course was in awe of this amazing plant's voracious growth. One day I came home to find one of the branches had manoeuvred through a small crack in a closed (!) window of the bathroom. So of course I did a plant journey with blackberry. What I learned is that this plant thrives on the urban growth here. The more the city grows the more this plant busts out. For many gardeners it is the bane of their existence. But here in the city there is an honoured tradition of the "blackberry season". It also bears these delicious fruits, which are hard enough to pick that they are not commercialised, but make great pies and jams. During this season many people can be seen along the streets grabbing for berries almost out of reach. So, in part, it thrives and controls growth, but it also boldly builds community in a cold urban environment, and provides sweetness.

One journey I visited scarlet pimpernel (anagallis arvensis). She came from a very humid hot climate with huge vegetation all around. The smells were amazing. There was a little wooden house with a veranda and steps leading up to the front door. I walked up the steps and knocked on the door, then stood down on one of the steps, waiting for the door to open. I felt she was expecting me.

She came out. Wow! She was tall, very tall, strong and large; she came down the steps and enfolded me in her big skirt. It was warm, I was home, protected, and safe; no one could see me. She had a Peruvian type of black hat with coloured ribbons and braided hair and a huge colourful skirt. I was enfolded in her skirt, safely moving; she was dancing and yet I was safe and no one knew I was there. (I had found ways of disconnecting and being alone because I couldn't trust people. I didn't know who to trust and who not so for many, many years I kind of made myself invisible.) I loved this lady, she was happy, soft, and kind. So we became the best of friends, Anagallis and I. Many years later I was helping a respected member of the community with his end of life care. He was a very soft-hearted person; he still had that sensual sparkle in his eyes. We would do drumming and healing together. One time I asked Scarlet Pimpernel to come on a journey with us. We closed our eyes. I went to a place where it was hot and the smells were the same as before. At a pyramid, I saw us saving children from child sacrifices. Afterwards he told me what he had seen. The smells and the environment were the same and he had also seen the pyramid and the saving of the children. With tears in my eyes I realised and remembered the powerlessness I felt when I was two and lived in a children's home and watched other babies and children being mistreated through the bars of my cot. On that day Scarlet Pimpernel was with us both.

When I first started learning PSM, I was smoking marijuana on a daily basis. I would get "high" at least three or four times a day. It was part of my daily ritual, as well as for those I was living with at the time, so it was a mainstay of our social culture. I liked how it made me feel more connected with nature and gave me a sense that the stressful things in my life didn't matter. When Eliot started talking about the dangers of messing with this "power" plant, I really had a serious negative reaction. From my perspective, he was attacking what had become my medicine, and my primary coping mechanism to get through life. During one class session in particular, I was really struggling, feeling anger and resentment. What had I got myself into? One night, I had a dream, in which the spirit of marijuana plant visited me. She was actually very compassionate, and explained to me that if I were to continue working with her there were things she was already taking from me that she would continue to take from me, things I didn't even realise she was taking but that were part of the exchange for her medicine. If I were not willing to let go of those things, and she assured me if I knew exactly what they were I would not be willing, it would be better if I were to let go of her. So, over a period of a few weeks, I reduced my use of her to nothing, and have never returned. In retrospect I could see what she was taking from me, and that was primarily a full emotional experience, which she had commandeered during my many years of use.

Plant spirits come in all shapes, sizes, and types. Some plants are clearly very special and have been understood as being what can be called God-forms, existing here in plant form, and at the same time in the spiritual world as divine personalities from distinct traditions. These types of plants are known all over the world where ancestral traditions, or their remnants, survive.

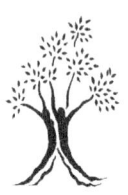

I was in Bali where I regularly go, taking small groups of people to discover the wonderful Balinese culture and ceremonies. I had to do a number of plant studies and journeys as homework for the PSM healer training. The first plant I felt drawn to do was rice. In Bali it's so abundant, it was growing all around where I was staying. I could watch it grow daily from my terrace. I made the appropriate local offerings to rice (rather than use the barley, oats from Europe or tobacco in the US). I sat down and drew all the different stages of rice, spending an afternoon chatting to rice. Then when I felt I'd got enough of a connection I decided to lie down on my terrace and do a plant journey. I went down to the lower world and ended up in a place where there was wild rice growing as far as the eye could see. This huge spirit appeared who took up most of the sky. It roared at me, "I'm not a plant spirit! I am a god!" at which point I thought, oops! The last thing I wanted to do was anger or offend or even disturb a god. So I said, "Oh, I'm really sorry to disturb you, I had no idea you were a god, it's just that I've been told by my teacher Eliot Cowan! He told me to do this, I'm just doing it for a course! I'm supposed to do plant journeys … I thought since rice was so beautiful and abundant it would be a great spirit to meet. My apologies for disturbing you." The rice god replied, "Too late!" since I'd already made the appropriate offerings to him and requested to meet him. At this point he gave me a whole lot of things I'd have to do every time I ate rice in the future. He also instructed me as to the power of the medicine that is rice and how and when to use it appropriately for healing. I thanked him profusely then I came back out of my journey and just lay on my terrace feeling slightly shell-shocked, and groaned at the time-consuming nature of what I'd have to do every time I ate rice, which is up to three times a day in Bali and even pretty often in the UK. Since then I'm a little more cautious and think more about the kind of spirit I might meet before I decide to go on a plant journey. There are certain things you do which on a spiritual level you can't back out from once you're engaged. For me rice nourishes most of the world's population and brings huge abundance and blessings to many lives. It's the last being you'd want to anger and upset, or it could create huge problems of all kinds in the area of abundance in your life.

Some years ago I was introduced to the Vaisnava tradition from India, commonly known as the "Hare Krishnas" in the West. I agreed to take care of some tulsi plants for the winter while their usual caretaker was away. Vaisnavas worship tulsi (sometimes spelt tulasi), which is *Ocimum tenuiflorum* or holy basil, as a goddess so sacred that they wouldn't dream of harvesting it for medicine. Devotees make offerings and dance around the plant, whose spiritual form is known as Vrinda Devi, the guardian goddess of the transcendental forest (Vrindavan) where the supreme goddess Radharani and her beloved (Krishna) are to be found. In order to gain access to this highly sought-after and difficult to reach realm, you need the blessing of Vrinda Devi. She can let you in. I quite flippantly thought to myself, "Ah! tulsi has a spiritual form. I know about plant spirits—let's go and meet this one!" and I did the usual plant study and journey. Wow! In the journey I felt myself to be by the banks of a river with trees to my right, and a full moon above giving everything a silvery glow. I found the tulasi plants growing and there was a woman standing there, a beautiful female form. I introduced myself and she looked at me and smiled—looking into her eyes was like looking into deep space, unfathomable black pools full of stars. I was filled with awe and also felt very embarrassed and foolish—I had not taken it seriously that she actually was a goddess. My immediate reaction was to apologise, bow, and back away. A month later I went to India and in the first Vaisnav temple I visited I had a powerful experience of spiritual ecstasy—I'm sure my relationship with tulsi opened the way for this.

The sacred plant teachers (such as tobacco, cannabis, peyote, ayahuasca, magic mushrooms, amongst others) also belong in this category. Indigenous peoples with intact spiritual traditions know of these special plants; science-speak calls some of them "psycho-active" or hallucinogenic. Such plants are always treated with the greatest of respect and their use is governed by strict etiquettes including the correct way to care for and engage with them. They are never treated as commodities. The plants are all understood as being powerful doorways to the spiritual realms. If you try to open a doorway without knowing the correct offerings, ritual words, and so on, it is very dangerous and usually leads to serious unwanted consequences. Think Fluffy the three-headed dog in *Harry Potter*, who needed to be calmed by playing him music. No music, you get eaten. It's nothing personal—you could be very well-meaning and be approaching the doorway for all the right reasons. Still, if you don't know the protocols, you're walking on very thin ice. As with all forms of deep shamanism, although the blessings which can be gained are enormous, the risks are correspondingly high. Fortunately the generous medicine of all the other "ordinary" plants is freely available with no strings attached.

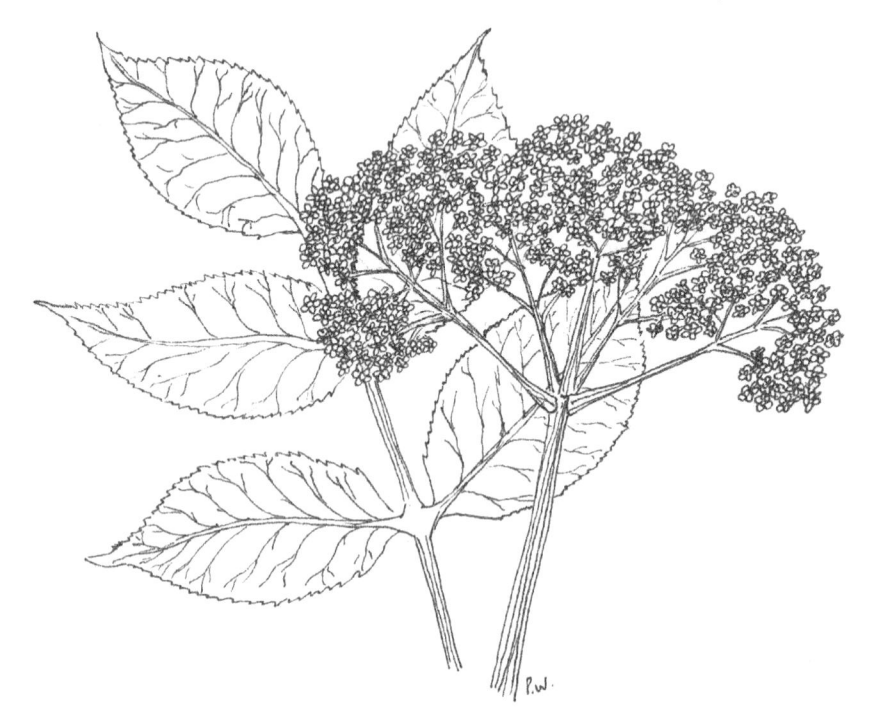

Elderflower by Pip Waller.

CHAPTER SIX

The healer's journey

Becoming involved with healing work is not necessarily straightforward. Our motives are not always clear, we are not always aware of many of the issues that drive us, and the path itself is steep and rugged. Healing demands that we confront our own reactions. A healing relationship involves both parties making an agreement to travel together whatever the modality. The call to healing seems to spring from life itself. In the case of PSM plants are the messengers of the call. Offering ourselves as healers in service to the people who come to ask for our help involves a journey of self-discovery and challenge. Working as an agent of the plant spirits is itself life changing and demands that we embark upon a journey over which we have no ultimate control.

These days there is a kind of trendy glamour to shamanism, which term can be broadly used to describe earth-based spirituality. Indigenous peoples who know what the shamanic path involves generally do not seek to be called to be such healers, knowing that the path is hard and steep, being essentially a life of complete service to one's people. Although plant spirit medicine belongs to the safer category of household shamanism rather than a deep ancestral tradition (which can cause great mischief if undertaken carelessly or without following the right protocols), it is still a path to true healership and as such requires a lot of sacrifice and dedication.

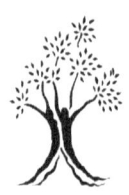

When I first started working with PSM I actually had a lot of resistance to calling myself a healer. It felt grandiose and as if I was making claims I couldn't possibly fulfil. I had been brought up with Jesus as the role model for healing and he could do miracles, so who was I? Along the way somewhere I became suspicious of this "little me" attitude and started to perceive it as an inverted sort of arrogance that gave me an excuse to close down from learning and got in the way of my becoming as effective as I could. There were times when not many people were asking for my healing help, and I would try to give it up. But always the plant spirits kept at least one person interested! And so I had to deal with my feelings of worth or lack of them and question ego driven motivation as in "I must be very important if so many people are queuing at my door and what does it mean if no one is?" Because healing itself comes from something much more mysterious than a human being could ever comprehend I needed to examine my relationship with mystery. After we have delivered our first ever treatment with plant spirits we are met with a huge round of applause from our fellow students and teachers and this in my case caused me some significant confusion as I didn't feel I had actually done anything yet I was being challenged to allow the appreciation for whatever it was I had done. Resisting acknowledgement for my efforts constituted the inverse of the blatant arrogance of self-importance my upbringing had taught me was bad, and was just as out of balance. Playing small didn't cut it. So the compulsion to follow a path that investigated true humility and service to my fellow beings was fuelled primarily by a stubborn investigation of self motivation and awareness alongside a desire to help make things better than I had perceived them to be in my experience of living thus far. This in some way explains my engagement with being a healer.

These feelings are echoed time and again from other people who work as a healer.

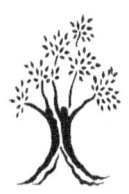

Finding yourself in a vocation or on a path as a healer is very hard, because what it's really asking of you is to make a commitment to your own healing, that of the environment around you, and your relationships. There is an ongoing process of challenge, growth, and evolution. You are often called to support people on a path you have walked yourself, to hold their hand and guide them. The people who need that will find you. In some ways that is an idealistic vision of a healer but it's what I actually see in practice. It's constantly changing. It's a hard vocation because you never really escape from your own process and there's a certain need for engagement with it that is probably higher than it is in other lines of work. There's a pressure to keep on working with the stuff that emerges, and the people who come to you will necessarily trigger and reflect your own process. It's a two-way street and that's what makes it so rich because there's a genuine human relationship. There are two people on a path who find each other, and in every interaction there's a challenge for our own process as healers. **Nathaniel Hughes, herbalist and founder of the School of Intuitive Herbalism, UK**

I really don't have any choice. For me it is about surrender. The more I keep my mind/ego out of it the deeper it gets. So, most of the work is on myself. There is always more to learn: from the land; the ancestors; the plant and other spirits; and my many human teachers—including my clients and students. It has been an awesome journey! **Michael Vertolli, herbalist, Canada**

I trained with Eliot because his book fascinated me and I wanted to be able to do the things and have the kind of experiences he described therein.

Becoming a healer in the first place felt like a huge responsibility, I was very nervous about getting it right. The development of it, what it has become to me, and how I now operate, has become a way of life; something that feeds me and gives me great happiness, most especially helping people open up to the presence of plant spirits and how they themselves can communicate with them. With hindsight I don't really feel that I ever "became" a healer, it was in me all along. I don't believe I am anything special, I believe that we each have a little something in us that when nurtured and allowed space to grow becomes something akin to a healer—a sensitivity that nurtures, encourages, and cares for. It is the natural at ease position for a healthy, well-balanced human, in my experience. **Rachel Corby, medicine woman and rewilding coach, UK**

Following the call to healing, however it may come, usually involves some sort of training. In the case of PSM, as in other modalities, there is a combination of protocols and techniques, feedback mechanisms and parameters to take in and integrate during the healers' training which also involves plant study, traditional diagnosis, the learning of the five elements approach, emotional and sensory discovery, and homework. The course at present involves eight weeks (each of seven days' duration) spaced out over around two years. There is an enormous amount of homework too—there is a lot to learn, the protocols are elegant and precise, and the understanding of how to apply these to individual people requires quite a shift of awareness. It is more than a healing modality—it is a completely different approach to life than the one we are all steeped in. It actually requires a dismantling of our previous orientation. Picture the caterpillar inside its cocoon struggling for its doomed survival as the butterfly genes, previously dormant, now rise to supremacy and destroy it. The caterpillar loses the fight and is literally liquefied in order to be reassembled as the beautiful butterfly. The caterpillar doesn't easily submit, just as our minds will do anything possible to create doubt and interfere with the sovereignty of the heart.

Cutting edge research describes the relationship with the heart and the brain. There are two-way control paths, both electrical and hormonal. It seems that the most healthful way for our systems is when the brain submits to responding to the heart's messages—this is described as the brain being entrained to the heart. Often, and encouraged by the top-heavy activities of our mind-driven culture, the brain dominates the heart, forcing it to follow instead of following its lead. This leads to disease. It is fascinating that one of the early signs of this is the heart rhythm losing its minute by minute changes as it dances in elegant nuances with the changing environment of our lives. Instead, when the brain takes charge a rigid regularity is imposed in which it seems the heart is less able to respond to circumstances. This mechanisation of rhythm can actually be an early sign of heart disease. Since the electrical activity of the heart creates the electromagnetic field enveloping our entire body, its health is key to all other body systems. This research is gathered and furthered by the work of the HeartMath Institute. We can begin to experience the dream of nature when we start to centre in the heart.

> **Heart-centred breathing meditation**
>
> *Sit in a comfortable chair and take a moment to say hello to yourself and allow your breathing to settle. Bring your attention to your heart area. Imagine that you are breathing in and out through the centre of your chest, where your heart is. Simply breathe in and out through the heart for a count of five. Continue for three to ten minutes. Begin to breathe from the heart as often as you think of it—many times in a day. The more you do it, the more easily you will be able to do it—just this simple exercise will change your life, improving your health on all levels.* (This exercise is taken from Deeply Holistic—A Guide to Intuitive Self-care by Pip Waller, 2018b, and inspired by the work of the HeartMath Institute.)

Plant spirit medicine cannot be learned by rote, as if it was merely a collection of information that need only be correctly applied. In learning to hear and respond to the cries of our patient's spirit, we are looking to find the key that unlocks the gate at the outermost reaches of the vast and beautiful gardens which surround the palace that houses a person's soul. That is the delicacy and the subtlety of it. We can't pin somebody down, as if we now know who they are, as if it were simple, and as if people could be categorised or stereotyped. Much of what we learn during the training period and afterwards must include an unpicking, an unlearning of the absolute dominance of our mental faculties over the experience of our senses. This is the cultural habit we are so deeply schooled in that we are ignorant of alternatives.

The healer's training course is rigorous and intensive and yet it is only the beginning. At the end of our training Eliot asked for two drums that different students had with them in the classroom. One was machine tooled, perfectly decent as a functional instrument, the other was made by the Sami, who are indigenous to northern Scandinavia. He showed us these drums and asked us to look at the difference between them, the way they had been made and how they seemed. The one was the product of a time dominated, industrial process that had produced a utilitarian commodity that would work to sound a beat. The other was an object of beauty and power, made from the skin of an animal that had been hunted with awareness, whose skin had been cured and scraped by hand, bound around wood that had been steamed and fastened with cleverly hand carved dowels. The skin was painted with images that described a process discovered through dreaming. Though both were drums they were as different from each other as a packet of crisps is to a lovingly cooked meal of home grown vegetables. In his inimitable style he pointed out that anyone can be trained in an occupation but it is only with time, perseverance, commitment, and the ongoing agreement to learning that we would ever get near to what the Sami drum represented. At least that is what I took from that lesson and it stuck with me: that training is only the beginning.

"Life is short, the art long." The healer's journey involves continual learning. It's common for people to come to PSM who have already studied other modalities as a way to deepen their inquiry into the art of healing. Because of the significant requirement to shift perspective away from the human-as-superior orientation, this can present an extra challenge in unlearning what we think we "know" already.

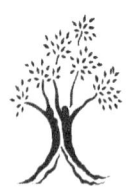

It was really difficult for me to learn to practise plant spirit medicine as I was already a healer in another tradition (herbal medicine), and like they say in class it's so much easier if you don't have another tradition. It was hard to separate them, and I found myself often falling back on my herbal way. The plant spirit medicine is elegant and seemingly simple but it's vastly complex. It's easy to put information in your head but the actual practice of it, in the presence of people, is the interweaving of the knowledge and being in your own emotional body in the right way, with all the questions, "Is this right, is this going on?" I had been a herbalist for ten years, so it was difficult not falling back into it when faced with all the awkwardness that I experienced learning a new medicine, to really allow the plant spirit medicine to come through in the right way. I would keep showing up to the medicine and it kept blowing me away. When I'd get insecure, I would see what it can do and that kept me going. But it's been a real struggle. I've recently made the decision to really fully focus on plant spirit medicine. I'm going to let my herbal practice go so I can fully embody plant spirit medicine, as I'm more attracted to, have always been more attracted to working with the spirit, in terms of this deep practice. Herbal medicine is brilliant, works in so many ways, it is excellent for physical stuff—but there are so many brilliant herbalists and we need more plant spirit medicine. Some things are purely physical, and you need to have a physical medicine for them, herbal medicine is ideal for that—but I want to concentrate on plant spirit medicine, healing the spirit, the emotions. **Monika Ghent, PSM healer and herbalist, Canada**

I picked up a book, *Plant Spirit Medicine*, at a festival. I was in my second year of a herbal medicine degree and I thought it was an ordinary herbal book. My mind was amazed by what I read—the plants are sentient beings! This reopens doorways that have been closed to many for so long. That was the beginning of my journey. I made a special trip to London in 2002 for an evening of plant spirit journeying with Pip Waller. A robin in the hawthorn tree on my journey was really aggressive towards me and shouted at me to go away until I was really ready for the work! Next I discovered Stephen Harrod Buhner, read his books, and did some training with him in Ireland. Learning "the language of plants" with Stephen was inspiring and strengthened my resolve to explore further. Over the past three years I have worked with Pam Montgomery who has also been generous in the sharing of her knowledge; how to cleanse and clear oneself with herbs, how to develop a deeper relationship with the plants, and how to invite new plant spirit allies to step in to bring healing. Pam is dedicated to her work and challenges her students to tell the world that we actually do talk with plants. I am now over halfway through my training in plant spirit medicine with Eliot and Alison and am seeing and experiencing the profound healing the plants can bring to us all. It is wondrous work and I am so grateful to have had the opportunity to learn from all my teachers. **Julie Wood, PSM healer and herbalist, UK**

I would say from early teens onwards my life has been a healing journey. I, like you, was born into a deeply damaged world to a nation of peoples who are painfully cut off from the rest of nature. I felt it as a deep wound from my very earliest remembering and so my life path has been one of working towards health and wholeness not only for myself but for all peoples and all beings: there is no separation. So becoming a healer has been a result of my own healing journey. The dictionary definition of "healing" is "the process of making or becoming sound or healthy again": as soon as I could see and feel pain in the world I knew it needed to be addressed, that "healing" needed to take place. If people are not helped, not guided to wake up to the reality of interconnections and their personal responsibility within it all, the world as we know it will be over an awful lot more quickly than we think. For the sake of all our relations, the beloved plants and birds, rivers and mountains, insects and animals, I am hungry to help our people. My greatest love lives outside humanity in wider-than-human nature. I love Gaia and I believe every being has a right to live, not just humankind but all kind. I believe that for all life to continue humankind need to be healed of our great illusion—that of separation; so that we can step up to the table of all beings and take responsibility for our individual and collective actions. **Rachel Corby, medicine woman and rewilding coach, UK**

Many healers, perhaps all, to some degree or other, are called to the art by the need to find answers to or meaning in our own wounds. I (Lucy) had heard of the wounded healer, and the adage "Healer, heal thyself!", and Chiron, as an archetype and the concept of only being able to go as far with our clients as we have with ourselves, and although they made sense I still felt a bit removed from it all. If I look at my life from the vantage point of now I can see its events and the way I reacted to them as lessons. There have been times when I have been tempted to give up or sign myself into a mental asylum as I felt in so much internal anguish and conflict. It's often been tempting to blame others or circumstances for how I have felt but getting to the point of taking full and honest responsibility for my own healing has enabled me to be more helpful to others as a healer.

Understanding the dynamics of denial has also been key and by that I mean starting to feel more open to how I am really feeling rather than a prescribed version that I think may be acceptable. In all of this both the plant spirits and my human teachers of whom Eliot is a most important one have been invaluable guides. I have sometimes felt the echoes of something ancestral in working with the plant spirits as if they have called me back to something I already knew but way, way back, and that the feeling of pain and deep sorrow that has been a continuous part of my living memory has made me persevere until I was healed enough to properly accept and commit to the path. Even today when people ask me about my relationship with plants I feel a need to explain that I am not a herbalist or keen gardener, I don't know all the Latin botanical names or go foraging for wild food but I do feel a deep kinship, a familiarity that is truly what has fuelled my interest.

A year or so after first receiving PSM and having embarked upon the healer training, I decided I needed to go back to the place where I was born and pick up a bit of my soul from where it was severed when I moved as a child following the break-up of my family of origin. The local church had played a big part in my family's drama and had been the site of recurring nightmares for me so I plucked up courage to lay the ghosts. The visit to the church was interesting. There was not a soul in sight and as I pushed open the heavy wooden door the eerie sound of the church organ came bellowing out. This sound had always been there in the nightmares. It was almost enough to make me turn and run but there was enough of the Hammer horror humour to hold me and I entered the church only to be slightly disappointed by the scale of the place. In my memory it had been cavernous, dark and shadowy, full of ghosts and torture; in this moment it seemed small, strangely banal, and insignificant. Walking later from the church to my former home, however, took me by surprise. There bordering my old garden was a laurel hedge and as I rounded the corner I was reduced to tears upon sight of it as if meeting the dearest old friend whom I had somehow been prevented from seeing. It wasn't as if I hadn't seen any laurel during the intervening years but I hadn't fully noticed it nor realised how it saw and knew me, how familiar it was.

This mutual recognition and the feeling of intense love filled me with an understanding of the security and confidence of rooted continuum that had felt so shattered and fragmented during all the transitory episodes of my life. They had been set into that pattern by the sense of abandonment and fear the painful divorce of my parents had initiated. That all of that could have somehow been held in the roots, branches, and leaves of a roadside hedge was miraculous and inexplicable and literally brought me to my knees. The combination of humility and gratitude I felt was like a complete balm after the tortured agonising and trying to work out why things had happened as they did.

It's not an easy path. We have to face ourselves, we have to face our doubts and the mirror of the outside world, the pull of the mechanistic, proof-driven world-view of our dominant culture which constantly pulls us from heart to mind. We embark upon a journey of humility and trust in a way of relating to the world that has been belittled and even demonised. And doubt is often present. It can be challenging to simply trust. As well as being totally useless, doubt manages to get in any tiny crack and inflate itself until it looks like quite a viable proposition. It seems to be able to get us in its grip. Doubt undermines decisions, causes confusion, prevents achievement, creates internal agony, and casts itself wherever it can. It is not the same as consideration, uncertainty, or assessment. It likes to put the boot in. So the healer has to deal with doubt and understand it to be driven by crippling fear, the cause and the result of so much that needs healing. Generated by the desperate mind it can so easily run amok, drowning out the wise, deeply knowing voice of the heart. As healers we learn to listen to the heart and its quiet, wise voice. Luckily the deep joy afforded by a sense of communication with the heart of nature is a precious and reassuring guide.

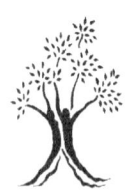

I say do what makes you feel the most alive. Sometimes I've thought, "Oh, I'll stop this, maybe it's not bringing any money in," or I think, "I can't do this, I'm not good enough, I can't get it set up financially" or something. But there's always something in the spirit world that says, "No, we want you to do this." This has happened all along for me. For instance, I had just done the plant study week of the PSM healer training with Eliot Cowan. It was a fabulous week where we learnt how to go and do plant journeys. Except I was feeling a bit overwhelmed and depressed. I was so ignorant about plants in general compared to the other class members. For example we were told to go out and do a plant study with plantain. I was walking around the English garden looking up high for a banana tree—the only plantain I knew was like a banana. But I was supposed to be looking for a little spiked leafed, fluffy flowered plant. I'd spent that week feeling like a fool, telling myself "The journeys are fun but I'll never be able to do it, I know nothing about plants." So I'm back in Geneva thinking "I may as well give up, I'll never be able to practise." I'm sitting out on a terrace at a restaurant with my two best friends for our weekly get-together. At the end of the meal, my friend looks at me and says, "Oh my gosh!" I look down and I'm covered with green wings, just like in *Avatar* when the seeds of the sacred tree all stick to him. My whole pullover was covered with 100 or so sticky green wings. My friends didn't have a single one stuck to them. Then I looked up at this huge tree we sat beneath, and I thought, "Oh! You're a lime tree [Tilia]—I do know about plants after all! I can do the PSM course." **Lucy Harmer, PSM healer, feng shui and space clearing expert, Switzerland**

I (Pip) have always wanted to be a healer though I regularly question what this really means. When I was five I wrote in my first school book, "When I grow up I'm going to be a doctor and give people medicine and X-rays and make them better." As a teenager I didn't like chemistry and physics though I loved biology and the woods, and the emotional help I needed was completely unavailable through orthodox medicine, so I ditched the doctor idea. I fell into herbal medicine through my parents' anxiety to get me on a career path—they had both been hugely helped by it. Although I have often thought of giving it up (and more recently after thirty years in practice, of taking early retirement!), I have somehow continued. Whatever life throws at me that makes me want to stay in bed with a pillow over my head, it also keeps reminding me via the gratitude of my patients that I am ultimately in service to my people, my community, and perhaps to the plants themselves.

I (Lucy) have found this path has led me to negotiate a huge amount of grief. Often it has been tempting to put this down to my own personal tendency towards depression or some instability in my own being. Some of that is indeed the case. Yet set against the cultural mores of our era, outpourings of tears, wailing, or indeed any strong emotion can quite easily have you medicated; but the times I spend in woods, on hilltops, by rivers or sea shores frequently elicit such forceful emotional expression and feelings of clarity and renewal I have come to understand that it is not so much just me that is "mad" but the backlog of unacknowledged destruction and pain that the land knows. We are forced to confront it if we start to open to it. Of course it isn't all about suffering and wailing on cliff tops but in denying grief and its cleansing capacity we make many more problems. As all the ghosts and shadows call to me to receive acknowledgement I am so grateful to feel supported by nature itself and the plant spirits in particular.

Practising PSM has been fantastic. I felt from the very first treatment I gave that I was doing something I knew, that I was remembering something. I'd have to say that I practised for probably the first fifteen years and people would ask me, "Do you work?" I'd say, "No, I don't work," because I didn't feel that what I was doing was work—it was so enriching and fulfilling both for the patients and for me. Then I'd have to say, "Wait, I'm sorry, I do work!" Working in this way gave me energy, joy, connection, and purpose. I've always loved helping people and being able to help restore balance for a person is an honour and a privilege. I feel very lucky to have work that helps others and is nourishing to me. There is nothing more gratifying than seeing people be able to reclaim their lives. I just saw a woman who had been unable to walk more than fifteen steps without stopping, and had paralysing depression. She slept fourteen to eighteen hours a day. She is a wonderful painter but had taken no pleasure in that for many years. While she appreciated her therapists and doctors and all they had done for her over the last twenty years, it wasn't until she began working with the plants that her depression lifted, her energy was restored, and she could walk without stopping. It may sound like a miracle, but plant spirit medicine healers see situations like this with many people. To be able to restore balance and bring relief is an amazing and humbling experience. I am so grateful to the healing power of the plants. **Alison Gayek, PSM healer and senior teacher of PSM, USA**

In support of the task of holding integrity within the complexities of the business of healing, PSM has a very clear professional framework. The dynamic for a successful relationship involves the client asking for help from the healer, making an appropriate exchange (payment), and agreeing to the process. Without this in place there is too much potential for misunderstanding and imbalance, no matter how much we may wish to help. On the face of it PSM looks like any other healing modality; healers have a consulting room, regular hours of practice, and adhere to a strict code of ethics. Healing is not regulated in law but successful graduates may join the professional association, the PSMA, Plant Spirit Medicine Association, which oversees continuing professional development.

Whichever way you look at it, plant spirit medicine is what it says on the label—a non-secular, spiritual path of healing and as such challenges us not to take out the net, display case, and pins, but to dance with the flittering variations of life just as the butterfly drinks from any source of liquid it alights on in order to keep its wings hydrated. As well as simple water puddles and flower nectar, it will drink from the tears of larger animals, juicy fruits, moisture from manure, and even rotting flesh. So as healers we are learning to hear and respond to all the various concerns of our patients without judgement, repulsion, or favouritism. In order to also read certain non-verbal expressions of illness we are required to hone our senses, opening them to receive the many messages that exist beyond words. Just as for physicians and healers in earlier times, one sense we rely on as part of the diagnostic protocol is that of smell.

> To open up your sense of smell, you may like to try this exercise in fearless smelling. Give yourself some time to use your nose to concentrate on what your nose is picking up. Smell everything and anything; flowers, leaves, rain, earth, wood, excrement, toiletries, animal fur, stones, furniture, friends and family. Try to put aside the judgement of smells as "nice" or "nasty", because it tends to close us down to simply experiencing the smell as it is. You may be surprised how difficult it is to not judge what you smell—this is a great example of how the mind works overtime to label everything and interfere with our direct experience. The more you practise this, the more it will come naturally and you begin to understand what it means to follow your nose.

There is so much more to training in plant spirit medicine than the acquiring of information and technique. As with all spiritual traditions, initiation is required. Initiation is the opening of a doorway by an energetic transmission that changes and transforms us in some way. The healing itself is really nothing to do with us. We are here on this plane doing our thing the best we can, and with practice and patience this opens a doorway to a world of incomparable richness.

My spirit guide took me through a doorway to a place of astonishing and indescribable beauty. I can't really express how awesome it was—it was like a magical jungle, a jumble of amazingly profuse nature, as if all the plants in the world were there—and not only their physical forms, but beyond them these spirits, from tiny lights to huge beings the size of mountains. Everywhere was an explosion of colour—ordinary and psychedelic, so many layers of existence in the same magical place. This was the realm of the Plant Spirits—I feel I have to give them capitals to express how incredible they are! On the ground I saw humans, very small, doing various things. I saw people I know who work in quite different ways, with varying paradigms of medicine, disease, and healing. It was as if there we are, doing our practical and effective but really quite humble things that we learn as healers in our various traditions, and behind us—backing us, what we are tapping into, is this magical jungle of energy just beyond what our ordinary senses are aware of. **Pip Waller, PSM healer and herbalist, Wales, UK**

While we are training we have initiation with a certain plant. As part of the initiation we have to travel to that plant and have a conversation with it and ask what it would like as an exchange. What it asked of me, which I thought would be very simple, was just to make a chocolate cake and offer it to the plant, serve it up with whipped cream and a bit of fresh coriander—I thought, "Why would anyone want chocolate cake with cream and coriander?" The first challenge was that I am gluten free—I wondered would that plant want normal chocolate cake or do I make it gluten free?! So it turned into this bizarre, complicated story where I didn't even know how to start, which is obviously the journey, right. I went to find the plant, drove up, I had my chocolate cake in a Tupperware and the whipped cream and coriander separate. I put the cream on and sprinkled the coriander on, and offered it to the plant. Then I drove off, but something didn't feel quite right. Maybe I had made the wrong cake, maybe the coriander wasn't right. So I called my PSM healer, and she said maybe it's because I didn't present it well. So I did it all over again. Made the cake, drove up to the same plant. This time I had it on this beautiful plate that I got in the charity shop, so it was more like serving rather than just dumping it. That's how I left it. It was only recently, five years later, that I brushed against that plant and I noticed its strong smell, it smells like coriander. I've been working with this plant for years and I never noticed its smell. I thought, "Wow, OK, they must be somehow related because they smell the same. The funny thing is that I had this real thing about coriander: I worked on a farm and I had to harvest coriander and I had real nausea, it nearly made me puke, so it was a challenge just to handle it. That has changed since: I love coriander now. But I thought it was really interesting and I can't believe it took me so long for it to click that this special plant in PSM smells like fresh coriander. **Loredana Kraushaar, PSM healer, UK**

There are many ways and various expressions of the art of the healer. In keeping with the living, breathing nature of the plant spirits and the healer's relationship with them, the twists and turns of our paths are as unknown and unexpected as life itself. Everyone develops their own unique ways of working and relationships with the plants, whatever kind of training they have undergone. What is demanded is the courage to keep opening to ever-increasing commitment to do what it takes to be of service, and to resist the temptation to ossify what will always remain a deeply mysterious and dynamic process. Just as in physiological homeostatic processes, balance is never a fixed point but an ever-changing response to stimulus. The way that we move, emotionally responding to our life, just as weather patterns come in as fronts and change in relationship with hills, mountains, and oceans, so we are required to fulfil the demands of the blessing of our life. We are called to move, adapting as we encounter obstacles, like the breeze across the meadow, the thunderstorm on the mountain. As we grow into our healership, we are constantly required to attend to our own development.

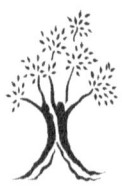

I have been a singer songwriter for many years so I suppose it makes sense that part of the medicine of the plants comes through to me as music. I had been working with the plants for quite a few years when I realised that I was hearing their "songs" more and more clearly and more often. I started hearing them when I wasn't even journeying. I would be going for a walk to the shops when I would start to hear a melody. "Where is that from?" I would think, then notice the holly trees alongside the pavement that I hadn't really paid a lot of attention to before. This started happening more and more. I was at the park with my daughter, busy chatting and helping her on the swing when I would hear a melody and look up and notice an apple tree was practically waving at me. I started singing the melodies into an app on my phone then: once I had journeyed with the plant or tree, I had the "words" and information/medicine to go with the melodies. I play piano and cello and used those instruments to provide the music to play the melodies. I've started hearing songs from the local rivers and the weather and sky too. I feel now that pretty much everything is a song. When I hear the songs of the plants and trees and all, it's not with my ears. I hear it physically in my body. In my chest and heart to be exact. I've realised all of my journeying is this way. I "hear" what the plants have to say in a very physical way through my chest and heart and I "see" the plant spirit in the same way. **Gemma Leighton, PSM healer and musician, UK**

Recently, with small groups of people, I have been exploring the plants and the elements through an embodied awareness of each season. It has been fascinating to see how for some the spring is a time of excitement and new beginnings, their body is energised and ready for action. Then for others there is a feeling of sluggishness or resistance and a wish to stay resting in the stillness, the safe haven of winter. I was interested to see how the falling energy of autumn is reflected in people's body and movement, how for many it supported a letting go of old habits and more trust in the unknown. **Anna Murray Preece, PSM healer and psychotherapist, UK**

Opening up to plant communication of course led me to understand that everything is communicating. The rivers, the mountains, the insects, the birds. And just as we can communicate and work with plant spirits we can do so with all life. It is my understanding that perceived disconnection from other than human life on this planet has led to the terrible state humanity finds itself in today. At present, I work with people mainly in workshops, retreats, apprenticeships, and individual mentoring (as opposed to treatments) to explore those lost relationships. Plants very much still guide me in the development and delivery of this work. Certain plants step forward to work with my groups; some of them are very regular, offering to work again and again with each new group, and with that my relationship with the individual plants continues to deepen and evolve. **Rachel Corby, medicine woman and rewilding coach, UK**

Now I take clients out into the landscape and help them through movement to connect to themselves and the environment. I teach them how to be in their own body more fully, how to relate to the elemental world by embodying it in their movement, and how to dialogue with different aspects of this world such as a tree, a flower, the river, whatever is relevant to them in that session. From the feedback I have received, clients are particularly enthusiastic at understanding how they can develop this process of direct reconnection for themselves through opening themselves up to the elemental world. Their experiences bring a sense of peace and well-being and have a profound and healing effect on them. This is a two-way healing relationship as the elemental world so needs us to take the time to stop and hear its own voice too. **Sarah Hyde, movement therapist, naturopath, and PSM healer, Wales, UK**

I use a method where I am completely relying on the sacred space where I connect and continuously deepen my relationship with my beloved plant spirits and all of the natural world. There are five aspects that are the basis of this relationship. Like the plants in wild places, the five weave in and out through one another. They are gratitude, commitment, trust, simplicity, noticing. The first has to be gratitude. A short prayer of gratitude to the natural world goes:

> Goddess within without
> How could I separate from Your waters in my veins?
> How could I separate from Your sky in my lungs?
> Could I separate from Your bounty in my bones?
> I am You and You are me, Mother who provides.
> Constantly moving to restore and hold balance.
> I am witness to your abundance
> Dearest Goddess, Beautiful Mother
> I pray in hope for our gratitude you deserve.
> That we balance Your Generosity with our Appreciation.
> That our love pour out to meet Yours in our place of prayer.
> Recognition, Realisation, Remembrance.

A very basic way that I demonstrate gratitude is my commitment. This commitment is an essential ingredient in my approach to healing with the plant spirit, done by being totally committed to spending regular connected time in the divine natural world, come rain, hail, or shine. I receive any guidance the plant spirits want to give me for my clients and myself.

Trust is probably the core of my relationship with plant spirit medicine. Without trust there could be no strong, healthy relationship with anybody or any being.

Simplicity is a fundamental ingredient in my way of being with the plant spirits. I simply fill my senses and awareness with the moment both in nature and in my treatment room.

The alternative would be to listen to mind. That would sound something like, "Am I doing it right, have I got it wrong, why am I not hearing, why are they not speaking, should I fast or pray?" Then I would be in a far, far away land from the land of relationship with the plant spirits' medicine and wisdom.

Oak has said to me, "Do not compromise the incomprehensible with your little mind. You cannot house this."

I have found nothing to compare with when I am feeling this simple innocence in nature. This is how I practise plant spirit medicine—how I see, hear and feel what the plant spirits want me to know about the treatment and the client both during the treatment and in between treatments.

My fifth and final vital aspect to my relationship with the plant spirits and their medicine is noticing. Noticing is a prayer to me in which I am giving my awareness to noticing, and I am receiving the gift of what I notice in my heart and senses. Noticing the plant spirits who are so full of joy that they can fulfil their spirit's needs to bring us towards a healthy balance where joy thrives.
Dawn Rafferty, PSM healer and writer, Ireland

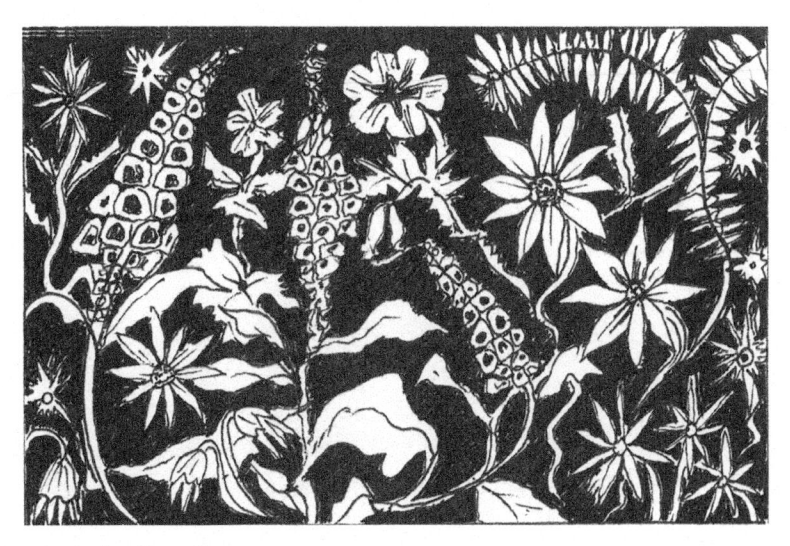

Foxgloves by Rose Perry.

CHAPTER SEVEN

Called by the plants

Indigenous peoples learn to listen to everything in the world around them for signs and understanding about how to live successfully; the wind, the movements of birds, the appearance of animals, the nods of plants.

> ... everybody learned that way. You watched the birds, you watched the trees, you watched the animals. You watched everything and you listened to everything ... For Indian people, everything is a message ... This was the way it was all the time. Everything talked to us. Everything was giving us a message. The stones, the trees, the birds, the grass. That's why we were trained to keep our mouths shut and our ears and eyes open ... The way we see it, the Creator puts his lessons everywhere. Built them right into the earth before he even put people here. Our job is to learn those lessons in the place we were given, and the way to learn those lessons is to sit still and listen. (Kent Nerburn, *The Wolf at Twilight, An Indian Elder's Journey Through a Land of Ghosts and Shadows*, 2009)

The plants have a way of calling us to their medicine. These calls come in all manner of cries, loud shouts, whispers, quiet hints, avalanches of coincidence, glaring or subtle, or simply manifest as life's twists and turns. It isn't a one-off opportunity but more of a drip-feed of developing awareness of how the plants take root in our consciousness and lead us back into our birthright of a fuller relationship with life. Often we may realise how a plant has been an important friend, ally, or support in our earlier lives. Without recognising it, the haven of a tree or a nook in the garden was more than a childhood comfort but also a necessary life-sustaining resource. What if the plants, as agents of a creative universe, were already knowing us and conspiring to help us at all times? This presents such a severe challenge to our minds that our materialistic culture labels it pathological fantasy, which goes to show just how separated we have become from the simple generosity of our living world, direct experience of which is implicit in all indigenous cultures.

I (Lucy) was a student of the Tao—a long-term tai chi and qigong practitioner, having studied with various masters, and sometimes taught others. I was a keen advocate for acupuncture but as life would have it never studied. I worked promoting creativity through arts, crafts, and performance but if I am honest I didn't deeply feel I had found my purpose. Drinking tea at a weekend qigong workshop I was sitting at a table with three acupuncturists. "Have you read *Plant Spirit Medicine*?" one asked. I didn't hear the rest of the conversation as those three words "plant spirit medicine" had become the only sound I could hear as they poured into my entranced ears with all the reverberations of a temple gong. Once home I went to my local bookshop (this was before owning my own computer in the days when Amazon was a river or a powerful woman) and ordered the book. It arrived the following week—and the next and the next, despite the order being for a single copy and apparently properly inputted as the shop owner assured me! I bought all three copies. I don't even remember the actual reading of the book except that I was hungry for it and this excited feeling that finally something that put together all the concerns I had for our human health, our relationship with each other, the environment, the plants, animals, and nature as a living force were being written about and woven with such elegant sense I knew I would just have to learn more.

In the early 1990s, I (Pip) learnt shamanic journeying from Michael Harner who pioneered this method of entering and working in what he calls "non-ordinary reality". I went on to train in some shamanic healing techniques. Through this I came across Eliot's book and was inspired to use the journey to deepen my connection with my plant friends. I confess that a prejudice against Chinese herbal medicine which had a very public face in UK, compared to the relatively invisible Western tradition, meant I never even read the whole book. I didn't understand the real power of his work—I just used the journey but still lacked a rigorous diagnostic framework within which to use the relationships I built. I didn't even know there was something crucial I didn't know.

After some years I began to share with fellow herbalists how to journey with plants. I taught a one day introduction to the shamanic dream journey along with wonderful UK herbalist, the late Christopher Hedley. The night before the seminar, I had a very intense dream: I was in the garden with a strange tree, small and spindly, flailing its branches around furiously as if in a big wind, though no wind was present. Although I felt afraid, I was drawn to the tree. When I engaged with it, it transformed into a black dog. The most wonderful dog I had ever met. Though I had never seen him in waking reality, he was *my* dog, a mixture, not retriever, Labrador, or German shepherd, but that size and type. His name was Magic. I fully expected to meet him in my waking life, and I actually missed him for a long time afterwards. Next day at the workshop we spent time with plants in nature, and explored using the shamanic dream journey.

Two years later I and some friends were looking for a property to buy in north Wales to run a healing retreat centre. We found a place on the internet that was very remote. We didn't even have the full address. Up the narrow winding country lanes people often get lost with directions and map. The day we went to look for it we went straight there as if pulled along by something. We loved the place, and went to talk to the nearest neighbour to see what we could find out. A black dog came out of the house, barking madly at us. Not retriever or Labrador or German shepherd, but that size and type of mix. His name was Magic. I took it as a sign just about the house. It was only later that the plant spirit medicine connection was made clear.

I moved in and immediately began to offer weekend workshops, and a few years later Eliot came to teach a healer training in plant spirit medicine that I was able to do because it was at my home. It would have been impossible as my son was three months old at the time. Really, I think the plants had earmarked me for it when I roamed in the woods as a child and made friends with the primroses, bluebells, and red campion.

They didn't give up on me though I was slow on the uptake in terms of realising the real treasure of the work. I now know that although there are great benefits in simply learning how to befriend plants with plant study and journey techniques, these pale into insignificance compared with the value of the full medicine, both in terms of receiving it at as patient and walking the path of a plant spirit medicine healer.

We are so used to thinking that we are the rulers of the universe that it might be an unusual understanding to think that plants could be responsible for our life's opportunities and choices. Could it be that we truly are one with the dream of nature? The evidence is there if we choose to notice it. The plants wave to us, nudge us, snag our clothes, poke us in the eye, look irresistible, enter our dreams, tickle us. They have so many ways of making their presence felt, offering us the experience that there is more than the material in this astonishing world. This of course is a two-way process. It invites us to listen to the offers of the plants whilst also making contact with them and letting them know something about ourselves. As in any conversation, it is give and take, and there is a process of assimilation about what is given and how we have received it. This is akin to what can be called "prayer".

Prayer is a conversation with something beyond us. At best, it is multi-denominational, non-prescribed, and open-ended. It is a dynamic heartfelt interaction. We can use this type of prayer to further our connection with our plant friends and learn to open ourselves to the many messages that life brings through them.

The plants have as many ways of getting our attention as there are plants in the hedgerow, forest, meadow, or cliff-top, and people are drawn to plant spirit medicine when it chimes with a need—to receive healing, to follow a hunger for deeper nature connection, as gardeners and growers, even to become a healer ourselves. The way nature works is so mysterious its messages may come from any source, at all different ages and times in our lives, often lying dormant since childhood until something triggers a germination. They range from a simple need to walk in the woods, through seeking help from a plant healer, to undertaking a course of study. Sometimes the journey to the plants is very straightforward, but often it involves a series of magical coincidences. Our minds try to put these kinds of coincidences into a box, to label them, to make something of them, or make them not be something. But what the plants do is keep us in the moment. It's about the feeling that arises, as opposed to creating a theory.

People usually feel "called" to become a healer. A calling to a healing path generally shows when some life situation creates conditions that compel us to take notice. Healers begin to understand that we have been following a thread already woven in nature's dream. Deep shamanic practice properly occurs within an intact ancestral tradition. For most of us this kind of healing calling is far beyond our remit. Working with plant spirits in the way we do in PSM, however, can be described as earth based or "household" shamanism to distinguish it from the deep shamanism of the rooted ancestral traditions. Household shamanic practice in the form of plant spirit medicine can be for everyone. Building relationships with plants and respectfully entering the dream journey with them is a safe and effective way for anyone who wants to deepen nature connection and is something we can all feel intuitively.

We aim to give voice to the plants' extraordinary variety of communication in order to inspire our own exploration of how the natural world will be calling to us, to *you*. To this end we have asked our colleagues, teachers, patients, and students for their stories. Remember, you've already been touched by nature or you wouldn't be reading this book. We hope that the sharing of others' adventures gives a flavour of the scope and encourages you to distinguish the true

Once again, make time to sit with a plant, ideally in its natural growing state outside. Make your introductions and offerings (see p. 39). This time, be with the plant and begin to do the heart-centred breathing described on p. 109. Once you have established the rhythm of your breath, begin to feel that you are exchanging breath with the plant—as we know, they take in our carbon dioxide as we inhale their oxygen. Allow the energy of the plant to enter and leave your being, as your energy flows into the plant. Notice your feelings and what arises in you as you continue this exercise for at least ten minutes. Any time you notice that you've become distracted, simply return your attention to the task. If you become aware of a question arising in you, listen for some kind of response that may manifest at any time, either during the exercise or later. When you are ready to finish, give your thanks. In the days or weeks that follow pay attention to what life brings you in the form of occurrences, dreams, feelings, insights, and coincidences.

messages that come your way from the relentless and cunning chatter of the doubting mind.

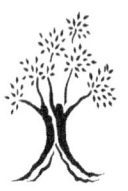

I absolutely felt called by the plants (to become a herbalist). There are so many occasions but the one that really stands out for me is the gorse at Arthur's Seat up at Edinburgh, back when I was still doing a chemistry degree, when I don't think I even knew herbalism existed. But sitting among the gorse there was such a tangible feeling of presence. This was my first experience realising that plants are *beings*. There's such a lot of gorse there, I could really feel the plant. It so happened that the room I was given faced directly towards Arthur's Seat, so I could see the gorse from 500 metres away. It was always there as a presence against a backdrop of a city that otherwise took me quite a while to feel comfortable in. There are so many little nudges and steps involved from here to my turning to herbal medicine. Linked with the gorse I experienced Findhorn, a place that has a very specific presence. Set against a backdrop of a fairly nihilistic absence of soulfulness, there were these little sparks. It's as if these things spoke of an aliveness that managed to penetrate through these layers of depression, and however depressed I was, I couldn't fail to be affected by being among those gorse flowers. So somehow there was something broader, bigger, beyond mind, beyond easy description or understanding. **Nathaniel Hughes, herbalist and founder of the chool of Intuitive Herbalism, UK**

It all started when I was fifteen and got a job with Neal's Yard Remedies. My mate's mum took on a franchise and she used to leave me there working for days on end on my own. I had access to a full dispensary and every dried herb displayed beautifully in jars, and all the essential oils that we could make into different blends. Out of everything that was in the shop it was always the herbs, the actual physical plants, that really appealed to me. So when I was sixteen I met a herbalist, Chanchel Cabrerra and I was inspired. I hadn't realised that you could actually be a herbalist as a job. I set about finding out what I needed to do in order to go to university to do that. Then because I was using herbs and working in the shop, friends and family members started asking me what they could do, coming to me for help. I learned to trust in the herbs and in myself from quite a young age, which was a blessing when I finally got to uni because I felt confident about going out and using them. A lot of the people who hadn't had experience actually using plants were filled with fear because of the way the university model taught herbal medicine. **Fiona Heckels, sensory herbalist and hopeful activist, UK**

The first plant I ever heard talk to me was motherwort (*Leonorus cardiaca*). As a herbalist I was learning to ID plants in the wild. One of the plants that I had always wanted to meet was motherwort. I went out to look for some. I was in a huge park in Toronto, I didn't know where to find her. So I stood at the entrance and I called, "I'd love to meet you!" and I was literally guided, a really long, twisty-turny way through the forest, and then I came to a patch of her. I was blown away. That was my first foray to plants actually speaking to me and guiding me. **Monica Ghent, herbalist and PSM healer, Canada**

I felt a massive calling by the plants themselves. The very first plant was a yew tree on the road protests in Walthamstow. I was a teenager at the time. I felt an unquenchable, unending sadness at the knowledge that this tree was going to be cut down to create a road. I was overcome with emotion. I spent three days and nights with the tree, sobbing, and trying to create some kind of apology. I continued to be part of the road protests and what I saw made me really, really angry about the destruction of our environment. This led me to my work—Sensory Solutions, which is the company I formed with Fiona, has the ethos and mission to connect people—or reconnect people—with their local plants in the hope that when they are connected they will feel moved and they will stop the complete insanity of the destruction of nature. **Karen Lawton, sensory herbalist and hopeful activist, UK**

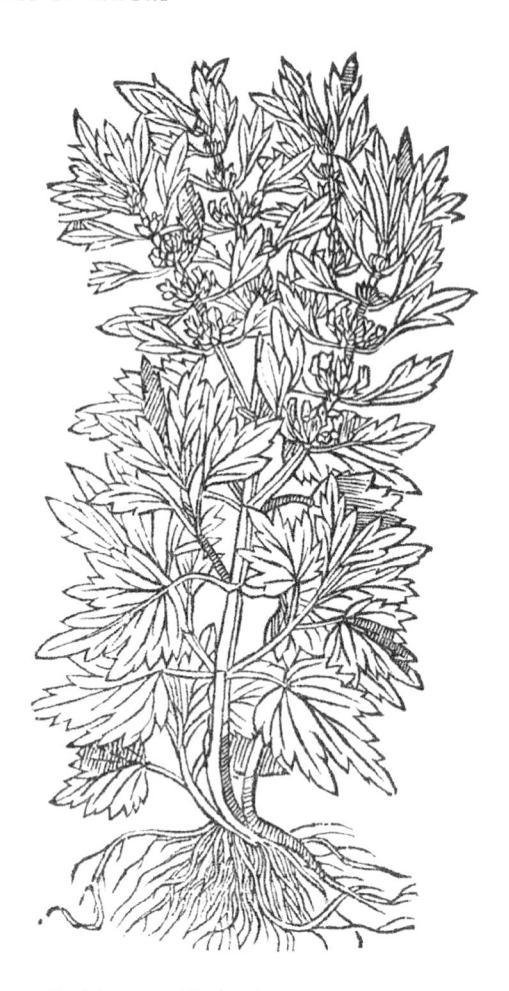

Motherwort from Parkinson's Herbarium.

My journey began when I was seeing a healer who said, "I'm getting something coming through … something birches, silver birches! We've got to listen to them." As she was talking I could feel a being standing next to me. The being told me to connect with my feet and feel the energy moving up through my body until it got to my heart. Suddenly my heart burst open. The healer suggested I go and talk to the silver birch, stand in the way it told me to, and that I'd know when to do it, as the birch would tell me. A part of me thought, "This is totally whacky! I don't know what's going on here but I'll go with it." One day I was doing some gardening and lo and behold there was a silver birch going, "Oohwoo, over here! Cooee," and it was just like that! I had to get through all this vegetation, brambles, and nettles to stand in a particular way with my back towards the tree and my feet on its roots. And sure enough, up pops the being. I couldn't see but could really feel her presence, an ancient, wise being standing next to me. So I'm doing the lining up, connecting with my heart and suddenly I felt her kind of step inside me—boof! Wow! ****ing Hell! It just blew my socks off. I was crying. I don't know how long I was stood there for, and then I carried on doing my gardening. I continued to notice silver birches. We've got hundreds on our hills so that's lovely. I could feel when the time was appropriate to hang out with them. I never had the same sensation of the being stepping into me, but I was aware of her inside me very often, mostly with her head bowed down, though on occasion I can feel her head is looking up and out. Shortly after that I came across the book *Plant Spirit Medicine* and it was like, OK, that's not a coincidence is it. I bought the book and thought it was amazing. Within days of reading it, up pops a Facebook invitation to a weekend on plant spirit medicine. I turn up there telling the story round the fire, and then I hear that this house where the course is being run is called Silver Birches! **Bex Syrett, Wales, UK**

I'm visiting a friend who lives in a little cottage in this lovely Welsh town called Llangollen. We were in a tiered garden up a hill up the back. My friend told me about how the neighbours were changing their garden, taking down all the plants and putting in wooden decking. We get up to the fourth tier of the garden, right at the top. Sitting there looking over the roofs of the houses, over the other side of the valley to Dinas Bran, Crow Castle, we were chatting. Then I felt an itch on my head, then a second itch. I started to scratch—is there a fly? Nothing was there. But more itches, and another and another, as if my whole head was getting prickled. It was oooh! So uncomfortable. I told my friend about it. When it was time to go, I finished my tea and cake and walked down the steps from the wonderful view after sitting beneath this holly tree and went to go home. Next day my friend called me and said, Simon, this morning they cut down that holly tree that hangs over my fence, it was under there we sat yesterday. Then I realised that the prickles were the holly tree letting me know something was happening, it wanted my help, but sadly I wasn't able to help it—but I do know that I'll know in future if another tree contacts me in that way I'll know exactly what it is and I'll do my best to help. **Simon Earle Huxley, SFC fire keeper, Wales, UK**

For as long as I can remember I've always felt a connection to nature. I played outside all day as a child, making dens from the bracken in nearby woods, climbing trees, building tree houses, constructing tents in the garden, helping my Dad plant and dig potatoes, helping Mum bottle home-made elderflower champagne and cough syrup every year—these were all of my favourite things! In my teens I became a keen walker and regularly went climbing on the local Derbyshire granite edges and camping in the Peak District. As a teacher and an outdoor centre worker, you could say I lived for the outdoors. In my twenties I started getting mysterious, severe pains in my hip. It took eight months of every invasive medical procedure going to diagnose the cancer hidden in my bones, and on diagnosis I was given two weeks to live. Fortunately, they tried a revolutionary stem cell bone marrow transplant and while recovering in my hospital isolation I planned my first garden. I don't know why but I had to and could think of nothing else. Since then I have gardened, planted, walked, and retrained and worked as a holistic healer and creative therapist and have, I thought, had a wonderful connection to the natural world. So, what was missing? I have known about plant spirit medicine for about ten years. I've had treatments, been to sacred fires (see p. 166), but something was holding me back from going any further. I wanted to become more acquainted with our indigenous herbal medicine heritage first. I went on a foundation course in herbal medicine and it was wonderful, I was happy! I started using it immediately and nature, it seemed, was abundant and generous in its rewards. Surely that was enough, wasn't it? Apparently not. And so I found myself on Lucy and Pip's introduction to plant spirit medicine weekend. I remember saying just before we did our first "journey" that I was already pretty happy with my life and my connection to nature, but if there was more to it than that, then well, bring it on! I didn't quite know what the result of those words would be, but what they brought changed my life immeasurably, for the better and for something that I feel deeply grateful for and awed by. Life has been richer and more beautiful than ever before and I feel "connected" in a way I didn't know was possible. It was as if the plants were saying "Well, you did say 'bring it on' so try this!" Imagine having a tail, like in *Avatar*—that you can plug into the trees, plants, and animals all around you. That's it! I now have an avatar tail! **Jo Jukes MRSS, shiatsu practitioner, artist and creative therapist, UK**

I'd been very sick from a spiritual experience in the north of Scotland. Very sick, disabled. This was the beginning of a calling but I didn't know it at the time. Six years later, I encountered yew for the first time. I was brought up working class in a city in Scotland. There were no trees. I was taken to the yew by a local tree surgeon; he was very keen to show me. We were drunk when we arrived there (I have to admit that). That lifestyle was a way of escape. It was a female tree, in East Lothian. Incalculably ancient. It had a chamber, an umbilical tunnel entrance forty feet long. You crouch low to go slowly through, like a birthing canal. Then it begins to rise up, finally opening up to an enormous chamber with the trunk of the yew in the centre. I had no understanding, didn't know what a yew tree was. I had no idea what shamanism was. I'd got to this yew by following threads; there was a dynamic that was pulling me and I found myself there with the yew. Coming out into a little moonlight in the chamber, I immediately became sober. I placed my hand against the bark of the tree, and a voice said, "You're home." That was the beginning of nine years and more of being healed, inside the cauldron of the yew. **Michael Dunning, Yew Shaman, USA**

I was looking for something for quite a long time. I didn't think it was herbalism because it felt a bit two-dimensional to me. Then I came across the plant spirit medicine website and my whole body went up in goose pimples.

Whenever I get a sign my body goes into goose pimples; it doesn't happen a lot but it's a clear sign. **Zoe Ekin, PSM healer, UK**

Many years ago now I had a strong experience with rosemary that was to change my whole life. I had been out in the woods on a cold, wet, and windy day and was feeling chilled to the bone. When I got home I was greeted by a huge pile of rosemary cuttings: my partner had been pruning the rosemary bush in our garden and had obviously been very overenthusiastic! I was very upset, I loved that rosemary bush, which grew just outside our kitchen door, and was worried that it wouldn't recover. I remember going to what was left of the bush in tears and apologising to it. I then ran a hot bath, and on impulse I added a whole load of the rosemary clippings to the bath water before I got in for a good long soak.

After this event I started to have some strange experiences. Every time I walked down our street past my neighbour's front gardens I would hear a little old lady's voice calling "Hello! Hello!" I could never see anyone in the gardens, but after a while of this happening I noticed that the sound appeared to be coming from the rosemary bushes. This was not a comforting thought. I started to think I was going crazy, but this voice kept calling me, and every time there was a rosemary bush which seemed to be shimmering and glowing. One time I was in London walking past a row of window boxes full of rosemary plants and I heard the voice again, so loud and clear from these little plants. I was on my way to a herbal medicine class with a wonderful teacher called Christopher Hedley that day, so at the end of the class, I went up to talk with him about my experience. He told me that he thought this was the spirit of the rosemary plant trying to communicate with me and this was "cutting edge" work, and that I should read a book called *Plant Spirit Medicine* by Eliot Cowan. I had told a friend about my rosemary experience, and she put me in touch with her friend Simon Lilly. My partner and I went on a weekend course with Simon and Sue Lilly, learning how to journey and communicate with the spirit of trees. It was an extraordinary experience which spurred me on to read Eliot Cowan's book. I loved it so much I read it three times in succession! Here was someone who not only had experienced the same phenomenon but had developed a whole system of healing with it. I was hooked! **Anne Lynn, PSM healer, SFC fire keeper, and Mara'akame, UK**

I read Eliot's book and it made a big impact so I was determined to remember his name. Many years later I saw that he was holding a course in Cae Mabon, Llanberis. It was a week in June which is a very intense time at work so I decided I couldn't do it. I quite often walk around the lake and past Cae Mabon, and it happened that I walked past as Eliot was arriving to start that week. I actually saw him, and it was like rubbing my nose in it, so I thought there we are. In the next few months my wife and I separated and I had a particularly stressful time at work extending into the summer. As things moved along I looked again at the Cae Mabon calendar of events, and Eliot was going to be there again in June. I thought, "Oh bugger, it's June again, I can't do it." Anyway, I was coming back from Bangor and I thought I'll go for a walk round the lake. I recognised a friend so we walked together. I told her about my disappointment, there's this Eliot Cowan course and I can't do it because June's such a busy period. So we're walking again past Cae Mabon and though I've walked past there numerous times and never seen Eric Madden who owns the place, this day we met him. We got talking about Eliot Cowan's course and Eric says, "Oh, I think it's a different format this year, rather than a whole week it's a long weekend." There was a bit of a "ding"—that sounds possible. Bear in mind I never take holidays in April, May, or June: it's a big deadline at work and last year we'd missed the deadline. This meant taking a day off, and it turned out to be a big decision. But I thought, there's too many synchronicities here, I'll do it. And it was great. The course came up the following year, I thought—I don't feel I *have* to do it, but wow I'm going to regret it if I don't do it. So that's why I'm now part of this plant spirit medicine healer training course. **Emyr Roberts, PSM healer, Wales, UK**

In 1999 I flew from London to Barcelona with my bicycle and everything I needed for a ride into the Pyrenees. I had my camping gear along with a bag of rice and a bag of oats. It was early summer and the weather was perfect. I rode north and then east into the beautiful mountains. I had no map and no plan except to see how the universe would look after me. I was fifty-three years old

and cycled with the same enthusiasm as when I was fourteen, so after three days I was getting very tired. I found a place in a valley where I thought to rest. I camped on the sandy bank of a small stream with thick undergrowth on the other side with a couple of conifers beside the tent and loads of firewood: an ideal campsite, except …! I was kept awake all night by strange noises that I'd never heard before—animal noises of some kind, so that by dawn I was a bit wrecked. While I was doing some chores by my fire that morning I was startled by what I thought was something coming up from across the stream. I looked up and noticed for the first time two quite tall plants about two to three feet high not far from me. I felt their presence very strongly. When I had finished what I was doing I went and sat down by these two and took a while to empty my mind. I then explained to them my situation and asked them for help (I'd never done this before, but somehow it came into my mind to do it). No sooner had I asked when I received a reply. They said: "You know, plants like us, we can't move around. We have no legs. Consequently we are completely at the mercy of anything that wants to chop us down or eat us or trample on us. The only way we can live in this situation is with absolute trust and if you want a good night's sleep you have to do the same." I stayed there all that day. That night I slept like a baby and next day I continued on my way. Many years later I met this plant again in the USA and identified it as pokeweed (Phytolaccaceae).
Michael Locke, plant spirit medicine healer and SFC fire keeper, UK

I was living in Berkeley, California in 1990. I went camping with a girl friend. We stayed in a little rustic cabin with no gas or electricity in a place named Mountain Wolf. One evening we were sitting on the top of a big rock watching the sunset, when suddenly I saw in front of me a dirt road that was calling me. I jumped from the rock and began walking that small road by myself. This road took me to a circle of oaks. I came inside the circle—they were huge oak trees. I felt I was in another world. I stood in the middle of the circle and the trees began talking to me telepathically. Each tree was a Crone, Mother, and Maiden; Baby, Rebirth, and Death. Crone said, "Welcome home, dear daughter." I sat down on the ground and they told or reminded me of all my life: it was like watching a movie with fast motion: my babyhood, childhood, adolescence, adulthood. I felt something coming out from my guts, going up and out, a lot of tears, fear, anger, sadness. I cried a lot while they were talking to me about my life. All emotions were coming out. That night was very cold and I was wearing many layers, but from the earth was coming a delicious heat which went inside my body, from my first chakra. I undressed because I was hot. I was feeling very good, calm, and relaxed. All the Mother Earth energy was moving inside my body. I was naked, feeling like a newborn baby girl. They told me I have a mission and I am going to do it with their help. They told me we will work together to help my brothers and sisters to heal and find their inner power, that I will receive the sign or message at the right time, I just needed to be alert and open my heart to receive it. In 1996 I moved to Asheville, North Carolina, and one of my massage clients told me about Eliot Cowan's workshops. Another time my boss who was an acupuncturist mentioned that she had been to a talk about plant spirit medicine from a man named Eliot Cowan, and sensed that I could do that kind of healing work. I knew this was the sign I was waiting for. So I registered for the class and my boss paid half of the tuition for me because her spiritual guides told her to do so. I graduated in 2000 as a plant spirit medicine healer and since then I have been offering this sacred medicine. It is an honour for me to work with this magic and loving medicine. Since 2000, my life has been blessed because I found healing and feel at home, thanks to the help of plant spirit medicine. I am so glad I listened to those oak trees and opened my heart. **Laura Leonor Sanchez Andrade, PSM healer and massage & bodywork therapist, Mexico**

Although it was my second outing to go and meet a plant, I was feeling a bit depressed because there were all these medical herbalists, pharmacists, and botanists on the course. I thought, I'm going to give this up, I don't know enough, it's not worth my time. I sat down to draw, which plant was it, a dandelion or something. Suddenly there was all these other little spirit beings, plant spirit beings, they sat round me in a circle: "No, you have to keep going, we want you to keep going," and I felt a renewed sense of enthusiasm and purpose. I was sitting on the ground watching this plant, dandelion, I was going through the motions really, not really doing anything, not even chatting to dandelion, just caught up in my thoughts. These beings were about 20 cm high, easily eight or nine of them, different plant spirits, they all sat round me. This was my first strong connection with plant spirits in terms of my healing path. **Lucy Harmer, PSM healer, feng shui space clearing expert, Switzerland**

The plants have a lovely way of encouraging us, keeping up their whispers and nudges until we hear them, continuing to guide us in our journeys. It's all about learning to listen to the voice of the heart that already knows our path. This is the central challenge of the work of healing in general and healing with plant spirits in particular. It is also essential to becoming fully human. Human beings have lost touch with their hearts as an aspect of the greater heart of the world. This is the devastating tragedy of our modern times. It is not a new phenomenon—the dire situation revealed daily in headlines and newsfeeds is the culmination of centuries of oppression and dysfunction resulting from this fundamental disconnect. The voice of the heart is not a sugary New Age positive thinking concept. It is the wisdom of deep knowing and all-pervading joy that underpins all life. By joy, we don't simply mean fun and laughter. We mean the peace and fulfilment that comes from real and true experience: righteous anger, appropriate grief, life-saving fear, compassionate caring, all have their place alongside simple happiness. To be able to feel these feelings, express them and move on is a hallmark of health, both individual and societal. So when we talk of the voice of the heart, it's not that everything feels sweet and easy. It's important not to underestimate the mind's capacity to fool us with enticing promises of comfort. This work takes us to our edges and if we aren't prepared to go to the edge, we're not doing the work. Luckily, this is what the plants are fundamentally helping with, or perhaps even orchestrating in their quiet revolution. With hindsight we can see that they always had us within their sights. The land itself is calling to us, and plants are the agents.

CALLED BY THE PLANTS 141

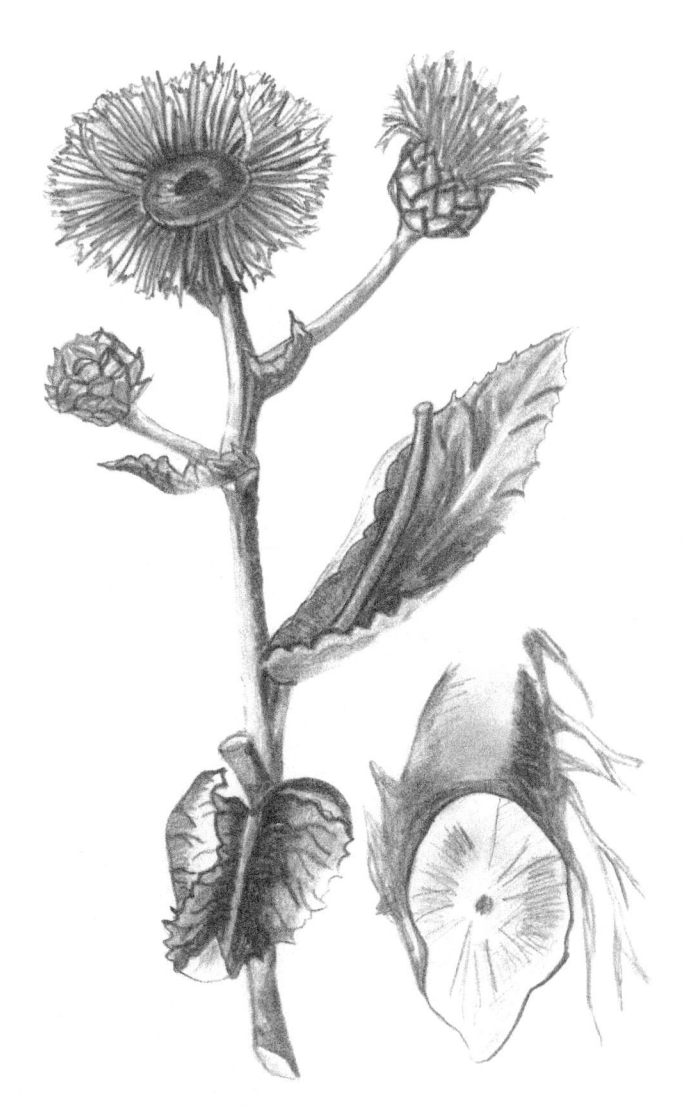

Elecampane by Pip Waller.

CHAPTER EIGHT

Journey for the planet

Why do we say that the medicine of the plant spirits is a medicine for our planet? Much of what is going wrong with human societies at this time involves a sense of being lost, desperate hedonism, disadvantage, exile, war, and oppression which have enormous impact on people and their environments. Politics are as polarised as at any time in human history; the divide and rule mentality is firmly established in every mind and heart, in every home, village, city, and country, and technology alone is not going to solve things. There is a tragic "Armageddon" within billions of individual people's lives in those parts of the world which are being completely trashed by the insatiable hunger of consumerism, and a zombie apocalypse among those of us in the so-called developed countries where much is invested in a multitude of addictions used to help us be numb to the rather grim state of things. And across the board a massive denial, as we fool ourselves into thinking business as usual is the way to manage a crisis. This further alienates us and the whole vicious cycle continues: the destruction of the environment, the continual extinction of species, starvation, cruelty—the list is horribly endless, and so many of us feel helpless to make any significant change in the face of this. This despair in itself illustrates how steeped we humans are in the belief that it's all about us, and we are the ones that must come up with the solutions. Of course we must play our part, but there is something about learning humility and our true place in the great scheme of things that is intrinsic to healthy change. Our central message is that we are part of something much greater than ourselves, and the more we allow ourselves to be touched by nature, the more directly we experience this and can be of real use.

Studying plant spirit medicine was not only mind-blowing in relation to what the plants were showing us and helping us with, but also gave the opportunity to start sitting around a sacred fire and listening to the wisdom of the resident elder, namely Eliot Cowan. During the day as a teacher of the medicine Eliot was extremely funny and deeply serious, strict yet kind. But the most compelling thing of all was to find somebody in authority who could be trusted and that was something that we were incredibly grateful for and continue to be so.

It was rare to meet a trustworthy authority figure. This is a sad indictment of our times, but nonetheless true. In the evenings during the course weeks he invited us to make offerings to the fire as a divine spiritual force. Permission had been granted for the use of specific offerings. This permission comes from an ancestral tradition with an unbroken lineage. The tradition we were introduced to originated from the Huichol people of north-western Mexico. Making offerings to the fire is an act of exchange that opens a specific relationship with the divine element of fire. Every traditional culture had or has fire as a central element. The majority of established religions also feature fire in their worship. As a doorway to the heart fire is the element of connection. It attracts and moves everything, from the atomic level, one atom to another, where fire creates all the complex molecules that make up material reality, to the love and attraction that brings one being to another and leads to reproduction in all species. It is the only element that reproduces itself. It brings warmth and comfort, cooks our food, heats our shelters, powers our world. Many cultures have very complex and involved fire rituals to invoke the presence of the fire deity but what Eliot shared with us was a simple ritual to connect with who the Huichols call Tatewari, or Grandfather Fire, although it isn't actually gender specific. Grandfather suggests a wise elder who has a strong and committed family relationship with us. Plant spirit medicine is one of his projects.

We would sit around the consecrated fire and sing, joke, and tell stories. As the night wore on a time would come when people started asking Eliot questions, not just about plant spirits but life in general, environmental issues, the problems of our world, relationships, and so forth and he would speak to us. He spoke with such eloquence and seamlessly as he intermittently puffed on a huge long cigar and answered question after question with equal thoughtfulness, clarity, and great patience. Sitting in the flickering light with the warmth of the flames as the fire ate wood it felt timeless and as if we'd been waiting all our lives to hear this level of explanation in this particular circle of humanity.

This is the gift that a true elder can bestow as teacher, guide, tradition bearer, and wisdom holder. Eldership is regrettably missing from our current societal make-up. Elders hold traditional cultures' wisdom and guidance. They have learned their art through their lifetime and carry the mantle of responsibility for the welfare and guidance of their people. Without them we are lost. When we found one, we recognised something singularly authentic.

The theme that ran through the spoken wisdom was all about the heart and the mind. This true elder managed to reduce the complexity of so many problems into a simple understanding. The heart is the organ of deep knowing. Our hearts and the heart of the world are not separate and the wisdom of the heart affords us a deep sense of joy, connectedness, and purpose that is everybody's birthright. This in itself was revelatory—it was hard to imagine life other than as occasional high spots with lots of punitive suffering! The mind, although extremely useful for certain aspects of our lives, is not supposed to be in charge, since it runs on fear. A life or a world governed by fear is in trouble. Our world is such a world. A helpful way of dealing with this particular challenge is to start to discern the difference between these two aspects and begin listening to the world with our heart. Although these concepts were not unfamiliar, never before had we been able to access this as a felt level of understanding. As we sat by the fire we experienced knowing this: it was not a theory or a mental construct.

There is no substitute for actual experience: someone could take hours and hundreds of adjectives to describe the taste of a particular fruit but when we taste it we know what it tastes like in a moment. This has always been the problem with following teachers or leaders. If at any time it feels like they are telling us what to believe in on faith, the urge to rebel immediately arises. Being guided towards our own experiential knowing is, however, a true gift. It doesn't happen all at once as all learning is ongoing, but tasting fruit is singularly nourishing and encourages perseverance.

There are many approaches to working on the world's problems—politically, socially, environmentally, and the teachings gained from the fire as one of these ways continue to reverberate and increase in sense: out-of-control fear is a massive culprit in the problems we face. We were lucky to be introduced to plant spirit medicine and sacred fire by a wise elder. As fantastic antidotes to fear they also open doorways to our own deep ancestral wisdom and make a priceless contribution to the imperative need for real transformation of our people and our relationship with the world. Of course they are not the only or the one true way. As we have seen, many fine healers are working with plant healing in ways that go far beyond the "plant drug" mentality into deep connection with the land.

I had one woman who had seen me for some thyroid issues previously. She had a little girl, had had no problems conceiving. Then she came to having her second child and it wasn't happening and she wasn't sure why. There was no physiological reason that anyone could find. We started working with daisy and looking at emotional bruising and any blockages. What we found was that her childhood home had been on the side of one of the road protest sites, and when she was quite young, but old enough to remember, ten or so, the sacred hill had been dug up to build a road. There were protesters there and she was watching it all unveil. This was the beautiful land outside her home. Without her knowing, it had created a deep-set trauma for her that she couldn't let go of, and it was preventing her from moving forward in her life. So using daisy, borage, and dandelion (which we make and call "drops of courage"), we explored the root of the issue with the dandelion, how we could move forward with the borage, and how we could bring back joy with the daisy. She did a lot of writing, went back to that hill, and wrote a letter to her former self, and also a blessing for the hill.

She reconnected with that land. What we made the link to was this beautiful fertile land that she'd watched being ripped up and dug and torn, that had become a source of great sadness within her physical being. So when we shifted some of that with the use of the plants it was incredible. After she did her blessing ceremony up on the hill it was almost the following month that she actually became pregnant. **Fiona Heckels, sensory herbalist and hopeful activist, UK**

This example points towards a connectivity between our individual (micro) journey and a broader and less explicable (macro) one. It illustrates the loss of deep cultural knowing and wisdom around our understanding about our place in the world. The desecration of place, particularly sacred sites, has devastating consequences. Surviving indigenous peoples know these connections with the rivers, mountains, woods, shores, weather, fire, and other forces and operate from perspectives that honour them with ritual, ceremony, and pilgrimage. Attending a conference of indigenous elders entitled Ancient Wisdom Rising in 2015 I was struck by the speech of one Arhuaco woman of the Sierra Nevada of Santa Maria, Colombia, who, when talking of the regular pilgrimages along the invisible Black Line that contains their country as the heart of the world, said to the audience that they don't just do the pilgrimage for themselves, it is not something separate, they make these journeys and offerings on behalf of all us humans. She asked all present to go and tell our people this:

> The "payments" or tributes we make on the Black Line serve our people in many important ways, such as in our traditional system of public health. It is along the Black Line that we gather many classes of materials and elements necessary for our traditional spiritual work. It helps with our own development in general because it represents a kind of bank where we find the necessary elements for baptisms, marriage ceremonies, burial ceremonies, and payments for all class of actions. Perhaps you are aware that our ancestral territory is very much affected and our sacred sites impaired due to Western development. We do spiritual work on the Black Line as a defence of our territory that represents all that exists in the entire world. This is why we call it the Heart of the World. We make payments to maintain the waters, the forests, the mountains, to maintain nature throughout the entire world. So from here, we care for everything where you are. (www.sacredfirefoundation.org)

Our rational minds may not be able to grasp the significance or importance of some faraway culture's practices and indeed may label it primitive or uneducated or study it as an anthropological phenomenon. But which of us if we are honest hasn't had a moment in nature where a certain awe or power has touched us instinctively? It's difficult to imagine an equivalent act of reciprocation on our own land that is concerned with the well-being of the whole.

The land has many homeostatic mechanisms. Human intervention backed up by our increasingly clever technological inventions has interfered with many of these, temporarily blocking the natural rhythms of the earth that maintain balance among many huge natural forces. One example is how forest fires control and rejuvenate the growth and health of the whole woodland. They have a way of being naturally contained by how the trees and undergrowth grow in relation with each other. When their natural occurrence of this cyclical fire is prevented, we can hold it at bay for only so long. Then when the fires come, as they must, the pendulum swing is so vast that the force of the fire devastates vast areas, raging out of control. This type of polarised human activity is happening all over the world, from arctic melt to mudslides, pollution-driven disasters and climate change. This is where the healing offered by connection with the plant spirits really comes in. Without us knowing exactly how, they are working as agents of the land to bring us back into alignment.

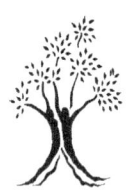

I could understand how we can journey to and meet another living thing—a plant or animal, but it was journeying to a rock that completely blew my mind. The implications of meeting and having a connection with a rock, a stone, the ground beneath us, the hills and mountains, that before I would have considered as "not living", feels different from flora and fauna. The timescale is on a different level, it's millions of years of knowledge and experience, our ancestors in a fundamental sense. Now when I look at hills I say hello—the hills are alive! **Becky Knight, textile artist and teacher, Wales, UK**

The yew calls us to develop new organs of perception with which to approach the elemental and plant world. We can't do that with the sensory nervous system conditioned as it is today. The yew is offering advice about how to be conscious outside a nervous system. To enter into a relationship with the yew is to enter into its consciousness. Those organs are not born out of the nervous system. Based on the healing I received from the yew, which gave me a different body to be healed from, my work is to teach people to receive this medicine. I work with one to one healing treatments with the yew, as well as in groups. Sometimes using cranial sacral therapy as the modality, sometimes with the yew mysteries—but always working with the consciousness of the yew. **Michael Dunning, Yew Shaman, USA**

I (Pip) had met many fine, and quite a few outstanding, healers in my time in the herbal world and on the medicine wheel or shamanic paths. For example, I was privileged to learn from the late Christopher Hedley, a true and great herbal elder who has touched the lives of many seekers of herbal knowledge. Christopher was a herbal wizard. I know I'm by no means the only person who first saw plant spirits with him, looking deeply into the hawthorn tree. Knowing Christopher helped me recognise the special quality of eldership when I met Eliot Cowan. So much of what he said hit a place of truth inside me. He is a man of absolute integrity, and keeps to a very high bar in this regard no matter how inconvenient that may sometimes be. Like Christopher, Eliot is exceptionally wise and at the same time not in any way self-important. Through him I learned more than plant spirit medicine—though that in itself would have been enough; in his wise teachings I found answers to many questions. I developed an understanding of the mind-driven nature of our culture and the enormity of the loss of our own indigenous ancestral traditions. I had been involved with the resurgence of interest in the earth-based spiritual ways of our own land—you could loosely call it paganism—since I was eighteen. Living at Greenham Common, I had been introduced to Mother Earth, Sister Moon, the Horned One, the Lady and the Lord. I learned of the elements, the special times of the year—equinox, solstice.

"We all come from the Goddess, and to Her we shall return like a drop of rain flowing to the ocean. Hoof and horn, hoof and horn, all that dies shall be reborn. Corn and grain, corn and grain, all that falls shall rise again" (lyrics from *She Changes* album, Moving Breath, 1997).

Following the threads of this path for many years, I observed the turning of the wheel of the year with ceremonial celebrations of the cross quarters; Samhain (halloween), Imbolc (candlemass), Beltaine (Mayday), and Litha/Lughnassad (the corn harvest in August), as well as the solstices and equinoxes. I learned how for millennia mass migrations of people had come to this island and all but destroyed the indigenous traditions, a job completed by the spread of Christianity and the association of earth-based spirituality with "devil worship". These terrible times culminated in three centuries and more of brutal witch-hunts in which innumerable women and men were tortured and burned or murdered in other horrible ways. The burning times destroyed not only the remnants of priceless ancestral traditions, leaving a hole that couldn't be filled in any other way, but also dealt a near fatal blow to herbal medicine in the UK since so many keepers of herbal knowledge were victims of that genocide. The legacy of fear and pain from these times casts its shadow to this day. It was from Eliot that I learned more truly what the ancestral traditions really hold, and understood that the recovery of our own must be undertaken in a painstaking and at times frustratingly slow manner. There is no quick fix in these matters.

The loss of meaningful and deeply connected communities that might journey together as the Arhauco people still do is perhaps a wound greater that we can fully understand. You need a community to heal. Without a community, you can't really be a fully effective healer and communities themselves need healing. This is known, it's been on the political agenda for a long time, funded and evaluated endlessly with projects aimed at inclusivity to combat all the problems of mental health, deprivation, and apathetic societal disengagement, but still the trend towards isolation increases. The fixes of our top-heavy culture can't effectively cure the problems that are caused by the same approach. The medicine of the plants has something completely different to offer. When we open to the fact that the plants are in our communities as healers, that literally changes our relationship with the place we live. Plants we pass on the street stop being objects and start being neighbours. In that respect the quiet revolution of the plant spirits is a movement deeply effective for bringing hope to the possibility of building real and healthy community.

Peter Wohlleben in his book *The Hidden Life of Trees* observes: "When trees grow together, nutrients and water can be optimally divided amongst them all so that each tree can grow into the best tree it can be. If you 'help' individual trees by getting rid of their supposed competition, the remaining trees are bereft." Who said nature was all about the survival of the fittest?

It may be that it is not possible for ancient and traditional systems of healing to understand or address all of our modern emotional and social problems. We modern humans are very hurt, living in cultures and societies that are often harsh and dysfunctional, even for those of us wealthy enough to have our physical needs met. It seems that taking sides and defending position has blinded us to compassion and inhibited our learning. When forces polarise, disagreement triumphs and the search for identity within this tension creates more division. We are currently seeing an explosion of identity politics. Paradoxically the seeking of freedom from rigidly defined roles and labels is creating an ever-increasing number of boxes and subdivisions. Most of us have lost our original culture, and struggle with the isolationist and separatist culture of the time. As Native American healers know:

> ... culture is the primary vehicle for delivering healing. The overarching principle articulated here, that "culture is medicine," means that connecting with one's culture has both protective and therapeutic value, promoting both resilience to and recovery from traumatic events. The details of treatment will differ depending on the cultural specifics related to one's culture; however, the principle of culture as medicine is the same across Native cultures, according to the healers we interviewed. Thus, indigenous means of treatment through culture may include any or all of the following: language, traditional foods, ceremonies, traditional values, spiritual beliefs, history, stories, songs, traditional plants, and canoe journeys. Connecting Native patients with their Native culture promotes better health outcomes. (Bassett, Tsosie, & Nannauck, "Our Culture Is Medicine: Perspectives of Native Healers on Post-trauma Recovery Among American Indian and Alaska Native Patients", 2012)

How can we achieve this level of healthy community? It's not a question of turning back the clock to some imagined time of perfection but rather a shift of perspective that allows for honesty and an openness to learn with humility.

At this time we are being offered significant help from our plant allies as neighbours. What does it take for us to listen, hear, and receive the benefits of that generous offer? The way we understand the mind and the heart requires ongoing and committed investigation. Nature wants to reconnect us to her dream. We are part of it and always have been.

Many people are interested in the great plant teachers such as ayahuasca, peyote, marijuana, and so on. This interest no doubt springs from a deep searching yet what we have come to understand, from observation, personal experience, and learning from elders about their role leads us to counsel caution.

> Some peoples were given sacred plant teachers as memory aids—doorways to sacred realms of knowledge, wisdom and healing. Some of these plants like peyote are ingested; others like the wind tree are not. But not one of them was brought forth everywhere. This is because, as we have seen, peoples are different. The Inuit and the Amazonian, the Aborigine and the Celt, the Zulu and the Mongol all have different needs. The ways of remembering are different for each. None of the sacred plant teachers are for everybody. (Eliot Cowan, *Plant Spirit Medicine*, 2014)

These powerful plants belong firmly in ancient ancestral traditions of specific lands and while they offer great healing they also can be a perilous route if not used appropriately and within the correct protocols. In the cultures where these traditions originate, a person would go only rarely to these great teacher plants, then return to everyday life and live the guidance given until the lesson is learned and the wisdom integrated. In our addiction-driven societies most of us don't want to do this heavy lifting ourselves. Culturally we are too used to taking whatever we can get our hands on; we don't take kindly to being told what we can or can't have. If we can start to understand the misguided nature of the human colonial imperialism of recent history why should it be any different in the plant world?

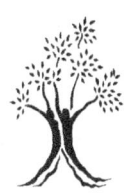

My wife had had breast cancer. She had conventional treatment for this cancer, then we did some research and we found out about cannabis oil. I made this for her. It was a very interesting process. I was convinced that the oil cures a whole host of ailments. It was advised that it was good to take as a preventative. So there I was taking it two to three times a week. But I found that after using the plant, the next day I would be heavy headed, less conscious. There was this fog, I was sitting in this numbness, and I knew it wasn't good. There was a trade-off. Later I learned about the protocols around all the sacred teacher plants that included cannabis. It made so much sense to me, I couldn't disagree. I also learned about alcohol, also sacred and how it can open you to picking up some kinds of difficult or unhelpful energies. I stopped using the cannabis oil (my wife had already stopped and felt much better off it). From that day to this, there's been change. So much change. I have no numbness, no numbness in the morning and through the day.

She came to see me for treatment in desperation. She was already seriously ill. Her cancer had spread and was virulent. Despite the efforts of surgery and chemo. This was a last ditch attempt at living. But she also wanted to go for the cannabis oil treatment that is lauded as a great cancer curer. As far as I had experienced cannabis always interfered with the treatments from the local plant spirits so I explained this. She still wanted to try everything she could and I sympathised. How would I be in a similar situation? I did not know. So with the agreement and understanding in place she came for a few sessions and always felt peaceful after the treatment. This was the most we could expect. The plant spirits could not take away what her life had brought her to but they gave some momentary peace, when that had been increasingly difficult for her to access. She died a few months later. At her funeral, however, I became aware of an immense feeling of awe about how little I know and how I need to be extremely humble and not assume anything about the capacity of the plants. In the face of death healing doesn't mean whether we live or die, it is much more mysterious than that. This was a seriously challenging perspective for me to fully grasp and of course would be unique to any person approaching the grasping.

Surgeon Atul Gwande writes:

> We've been wrong about what our job is in medicine. We think our job is to ensure health and survival. But really it is larger than that. It is to enable well-being. And well-being is about the reasons one wishes to be alive. (Atul Gawande, *Being Mortal: Medicine and What Matters in the End*, 2014)

The deep healing offered by our local plants is revolutionary in the deepest sense of the word, having as it does the ability to call us home to ourselves. It's a local medicine, rooted in where we live, where our patients live, where the plants live and grow. The well-being of one is the well-being of the other.

An especially beautiful aspect of PSM is its pure zest for life. Lacking in the doubt, guilt, shame, and despondency that have infected us Western first world humans for who knows how long, it helps us realise something deeply joyful. This is not to say that challenge, loss, disappointment, and difficulties all magically disappear. They don't. That isn't life on this earth. Martin Prechtel describes a similar perspective following a massive earthquake in Guatemala:

> But that day as we all sat together in Cuchumaquic, these starving people and this leveled land were for me the first tangible living example of something that had been at the core of everything I and thousands of other 1960s kids ... had been spiritually swimming towards ... I came to realize that these three hundred dusty people were not a backwards-looking dejected people that needed my help and a revolution, but were the vivid manifestation of the live flowering of what in English I can only call Peace. (Martin Prechtel, *An Unlikely Peace in Cuchumaquic*, 2011)

How can we hold a vision of wholeness for the world where joy and peace are not only a birthright but lived out? A place to start is with our own individual vision of wholeness. Often when faced with the enormity of the problems of the world, we can get lost in solution finding or hopelessness and the feeling that there just isn't a big enough sticking plaster. We are part of the same web of life as the plant spirits, and we are not on our own trying to repair it. It is made up of everything. Feeling separate causes the pain, as if we are alone trying to do something impossible. It is difficult seeing so much overwhelming need and how far into chaotic destruction everything has fallen.

There's a simplicity in joining things up, bringing things closer; it's what we need, and this is absolutely what the plants are offering—they are the join-up between nature—the earth, the water, the sun, the wind, and the humans. All around us, the land and the plants that grow from it are describing an extraordinary pattern of interdependency, a dance of mutual exchange. However it started, we humans became so engrossed with ourselves, as in the story of Narcissus and countless other cultural archetypes of self-absorption, that we simply forgot and in that forgetting have lost our way. The doorway to remembering hasn't gone away, the spirits of nature can guide us there but just how much help is necessary does first need to be recognised. For many of us this is a journey in itself. Asking for help in coming to terms with our grief, our anger, our desire to be useful, our fears and joys or lack of them is part of the healing equation. It acknowledges responsibility for our part in the whole.

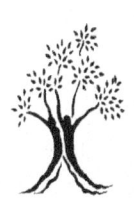

Each and every plant seems to have its own message. If you truly walk in the wilds and let the plants open up and speak to you, I do believe that they have a way of taking you on a journey through life, and you're never alone once the hedgerow opens up to you. **Fiona Heckels, sensory herbalist and hopeful activist, UK**

I do feel the landscape where we live in west Wales has been guiding me for a long time. I have struggled for years to keep "doing" in it. Meanwhile the land has been challenging me, often through illness, to stop and listen and receive it on a very deep level. When I enter this more intuitive, feminine way of being there is a flow and ease to the tasks I do because I am working with the energy of the land rather than trying to impose my will onto it. **Sarah Hyde, movement therapist, naturopath, and PSM healer, Wales, UK**

One of my most memorable journeys was with European goldenrod, a yellow thing that's often in damp places. It was on Dartmoor I found it. It was my birthday, September, and I knew where it was. I drove to it, found it OK: it was all along one bank. I did a study of it, drawing it and eating it. I introduced myself, "I'm a student of plant spirit medicine, would you like to tell me something about your medicine?" and made offerings. It was all going OK, ticketyboo. Then my plan was I'd go back to where I was staying, with my then girlfriend, and I'd do the journey before celebrating my birthday. It was all arranged. I knew something wasn't quite right, I had a kind of feeling. Then on the way back, it was about seven miles over the hills, I ran out of petrol; this was like 900 feet up, it was cold, I knew it would get dark, so I kind of still felt under the spell of this plant, like it was in me and I had to accept that everything that happened would be part of my experience with the plant, I just had to surrender to that. So I think the third car that came along gave me a lift to get petrol at the petrol station at Ashburton, and then somehow I quickly got a lift back, and both of the people who gave me lifts loved Dartmoor, their lives were intertwined. One of them just drove over Dartmoor to get back from work, but his whole way of being was to just enjoy that journey and take in the landscape. The other one was doing fencing or something like that, more rugged, he felt so connected to the moor, and I felt I'm meeting this plant through the people in the area, that's fantastic. So I got the petrol back to the car, he went off, the second driver, and the car still wouldn't start. So I had to phone the breakdown people. And it was before I had a mobile phone. I had to walk to the Two Bridges Hotel to use their phone. As I was standing at the bar, and it was now dark and a bit cold and rainy, there was a guy playing honkytonk piano, beautiful piano, and ladies in their 1940s finery, they were very old ladies just dressed up, and gentlemen. They weren't really dancing, they were just having a nice nosh, and this piano playing and the glittering chandeliers and it was like going back in time, and I thought "This is really nice, this is beautiful. What's the plant saying to me now?" It was all from the plant; the whole thing of getting the fuel, waiting for the breakdown people to come, and having to witness this music and their beautiful time together. Then the breakdown guy picked me up from the pub and drove to the car, got it started. I drove home and did another journey to the plant. But the actual way the universe put those experiences of connecting with those different people on Dartmoor, the sense of watery-ness, the rain, the dark, going inside this lovely cave with people enjoying themselves in a kind of timeless setting, the journey didn't really matter, it had all taken care of itself in my experience of the plant. **Peter Neumann, herbalist, candle and incense maker, and PSM healer, UK**

Of all my precious plant spirit allies, hawthorn is my best friend and chief advisor. The first one that ever called me to him started spouting poetry, simple poetry helping me to notice and to deepen my awareness of myself and my environment. A number of summers ago—thankfully, I have long since lost count, I visited hawthorn to cry on his shoulder so to speak. I needed his wisdom and comfort. I completely trusted that he was going to help me. I could hear the words I was using, and knew they weren't healthy but I was so distraught that I couldn't get past them. I was stuck on, "Look what he did to me." My dear old precious hawthorn calmly replied, "And did you do anything to yourself?" He softly continued in these words as though it was my own heart that was speaking to me.

> Lay down to rest
> Lay down your labour
> And your armour
> Lay bare this heart
> And confess disregard for my whispers and calls
> Disrespect for the needs I deserved
> Embrace your sorrow
> Come to peace

And love me again
Love me more than before
And we'll dream
          Dawn Rafferty, PSM healer and writer, Ireland

When I was studying plant spirit medicine I really struggled to pass my pulse exam which is a very important diagnostic tool. I had finished the course but couldn't practise PSM because of this. I was, however, getting clients coming to see me for "hole in one" treatments with mugwort to help with back pain and other structural problems. Not only were clients experiencing relief with their structural problems but they were also finding things were shifting in their life on a mental and spiritual level as well. I was developing a strong bond with mugwort because for a good while it was the only plant I was working with. Mugwort started to give me advice for my clients that I would recount to them. It seemed to be relevant and pertinent advice, even if I did struggle for a while to fully trust that this was mugwort speaking to me and not my mind making it all up! I had a session with a very pregnant and overdue client one day and mugwort asked me to sing her a song in the treatment. I do not have a good singing voice, and am very shy about singing in front of people, but I sang the song to my client because mugwort asked me to. The client burst into tears and told me the song was very personal to her and had brought up a lot of emotion which really shifted something for her. Her baby was born a couple of days later. After that experience I was able to fully trust that it was mugwort I was hearing and that all I had to do was get my own mind out of the way with its doubts and fears and just become a conduit for mugwort's healing energy. I passed my pulse exam finally and have been practising PSM for a good many years now but I always reserve time to sit by the fire and quieten my mind in the treatment sessions so that I can hear mugwort's advice for my client. I often give mugwort plants to my clients if they ask for one, and they report that they feel safe and protected with mugwort growing in their garden. These mugwort plants seem to reproduce prolifically so my clients are giving plants to their friends and families. I like the idea that in a small way I am part of the mugwort revolution! **Anne Lynn, PSM healer, SFC fire keeper, and Mara'akame, UK**

However you may view the evolution of our planet and its bountiful life forms, from a Darwinian/scientific Western perspective, from an indigenous one, or simply as a human getting through the days, our coexistence with plants cannot be disputed. We are all living here together. The plant spirits are so very effective at the kind of joining up of the dots that is urgently needed as we try desperately to address all the pressing issues of the day. It's almost as if we humans are drowning in the quicksand of our own nonsense and the plants are offering their help to pull us out. Will we take it and let them, or keep asserting our superiority and try to pull them in with us?

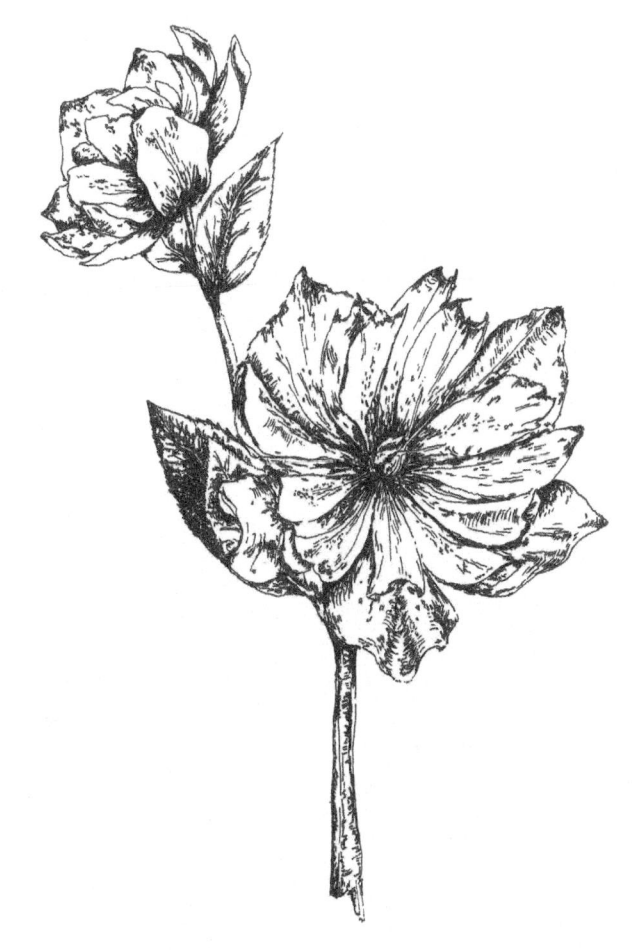

Hellebore by Lily Tonkin Wells.

CHAPTER NINE

The onward journey—how the plants direct us

When we engage the help of the plant spirits, there is a way that things seem to work out. The plants are joining things up, they make connections, they darn the metaphorical holes in our old socks. On a physical level, plants connect via a vast underground network of fungal threads, the mycelium web, through which they communicate with each other on all sorts of important matters such as sharing nutrients and information. They can even spread toxic chemicals through the network to deter unwelcome plants. Perhaps the plant spirits somehow use this mycelial network to spiritually communicate or maybe there is not really a distinction. However it's done, the plants are expert networkers. They open up doorways. The web of life gets healed. The more people move fluidly in their own flow, the more balanced our societies are.

The doorways the plants open for us are as varied as our needs. For one the plant spirits' blessings might help them feel more alive and fulfilled in their work, a bored nursery nurse for instance might find a deep appreciation supporting young children to learn. For another a calling to a deep ancestral tradition might be the way to fulfil his or her purpose. Whether we are a worn-out mum beginning to feel more supported in her often undervalued role or a creative writer in a dead-end job needing to find the courage to be himself and write again, the medicine of the plant spirits helps to unlock the aliveness that transforms everyday life. From making all-round better decisions to finding one's own true path in life, however humble, the plant spirits help us.

However it is that they are touching us, it is always in keeping with their deep knowing of us; they intuit just what we need the most to grow and become ourselves and find fulfilment—become our own vision of wholeness. After all, they are experts at growing in all kinds of circumstances, and still finding ways to flourish, to sprout, grow, blossom, and fruit. Just as the mycelial network sends communication between the plants, so the plant spirits facilitate us to join with our soul's calling even across cultures. The stories in this chapter tell of some of the ways that plant spirit medicine has worked to call people to paths of lifelong commitment: as fire keepers, weather workers, traditional shamanic healers, and those on other sacred pilgrimage paths.

Very few indigenous peoples have escaped the interruption or even complete destruction of their ancestral healing traditions by colonising forces. The Huichols, being a mountain people, are one of the rare few whose lineage remains unbroken and fully intact.

> The teachings are for all, not just for Indians ... The white people never wanted to learn before ... Now they have a different understanding, and they do want to learn. We are all children of God. The tradition is open to anyone who wants to learn. But who really wants to learn? (Don Jose Matsuwa, Huichol, 1989)

Eliot himself is an example of someone who experienced a deep calling to learn, and followed it determinedly. After many years of apprenticeship he was initiated as a *Mara'akame*, a shaman in the Mexican Huichol tradition, then after many more years he was initiated as a *Tsaurirrikame*, qualified to guide others on that path. The following offerings are from some of his apprentices and initiates.

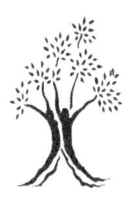

I felt called to medicine to help people, to really see people and help a deeper place in them, and I had doctors who were mentors in that. While studying as a doctor in medical school, I saw the gifts and limitations of Western medicine. I began to see how people reach dead ends even while living, and the magnitude of depression, chronic illness, failed marriages, violence, confusions, dissatisfaction, weird illnesses that no one can help, has only increased. I realised that the medicine I was learning didn't have much to offer people in these conveyor belt situations. I kept the following question on my plate, "What might help people move beyond this dead end?"

By the age of twenty-eight, I was a medical doctor and furthering my training in family medicine when I became pregnant. At three months I was throwing up in the waste cans during morning medical rounds. I learned that one of my patients with HIV/AIDS needed an operation. He was alone, terrified, and fighting for his life. I couldn't bear to hand him off to a group of surgeons who didn't know him as a person. I offered to scrub in and assist in the surgery. Little did I know how that decision would change the course of my life. During the operation, I was accidentally stuck with a needle. This was 1990, people were dying of AIDS right and left. There was a lot of fear and confusion. The response to the accident was prompt yet panicked. After immediately washing my hands with bleach, I was advised by the infectious disease specialist, "We're really sorry but given you are pregnant you have two choices—either have an abortion or take a special medication called AZT within one hour. This might help prevent transmission of the HIV virus to your unborn baby but we don't know for sure, and we don't know if there are any side effects."

I was in shock, anger, fear, and grief all combined into one frozen ball. What does one do when faced with untenable choices? I called for my husband and cried, then we held each other and got really quiet. I mean really quiet like a surrendering where there was no emotion or thought about what should we do. I began to hear something—a voice, a teaching, guidance. "Everything is going to be alright, I'm going to be alright (not I Lisa, but I the baby). You just take care of yourselves." The voice also said, "The most important job you'll have is being a mother." This place of quiet surrender opened to listening and exchange. Rather than deciding between taking medicine or terminating my pregnancy, I suddenly saw a different path. This new path, however, was a bit of a riddle not necessarily to solve but to unpack and discover. The guidance we received illuminated the fear based culture we are marinating in, which I had been calling the conveyor belt leading people to a dead end way of living. It carried a sense of uncertainty and fear yet was mysterious and exciting—I knew it would require courage. What did it mean to take care of ourselves? What did it mean to be a mother? And what does everything being alright look or feel like? It became clear that working while being a mom to a newborn was not a good way to take care of ourselves or value the job of mothering. "Alright" didn't mean that I or my baby weren't going to get HIV or even die. It meant we would have what we needed to face situations that life brings. The whole notion of expectations and outcome were up for reconsideration. Through grace and the support of my husband, I decided to leave my residency training and focus on being a mother. My mentors were not supportive. They had juggled it all, why couldn't I? One even told me I was making the worst mistake of my life. This made me feel like everything I had done was a waste and that I was going to live a failed life.

Going against the grain was scary but there I discovered courage and freedom. Soon after that decision I saw a flier for a course and met my first plant teacher, Dr Tieraona Low Dog. I became steeped in herbal medicine. Of all the teachings she shared, the one that was seeded in me was a simple statement she made almost in passing. She said that her grandfather worked with just five plants. Through deep friendship with them, the plants were very generous with their gifts, so he was able to help a lot of people. I kept this precious question inside my heart for five years, "How does one make friends with plants in such a way that they come and help our people who desperately need help?" During those years, I immersed myself in the wonderment and exhaustion of mothering, working part-time as a general physician and with plant medicines and maintained a very simple practice of Buddhist meditation.

When my children were of an age I knew it was time to complete my medical training. An old friend, also a doctor, told me, "I just completed this course called plant spirit medicine with Eliot Cowan and it turned my world upside down." I said, "Where do I sign up?" I knew nothing about him or it but I trusted my dear friend: she knew my heart. During the first hour of class, I knew I was in the right place when Eliot began to talk about friendship with plants, and reminded us that we were all there out of care and concern for our people. To help will require sacrifice just like the plants make sacrifices to help our people. That is the way the world is made—exchange and relationship. I was searching my whole life for someone to recognise that which had called me from the beginning and here it was. Soon after becoming a PSM healer I was surprised to be called to become an apprentice on the Huichol traditional path, to become a Mara'akame (traditional healer and ritual leader). During my fifteen year apprenticeship, I maintained a practice as a family physician and PSM healer focusing on pregnancy, birth, and care of children. When I began offering healing as a Mara'akame the plant spirits were singing more loudly in a way. They were reminding me of our deep abiding friendship and waking something up in me that gave me confidence to set them aside for a while. I had been working so intimately with them for almost twenty years so there was some grief, though I don't feel like it's saying goodbye, it's just that to deepen in this Huichol traditional medicine I need to devote myself completely to it—kind of like when I was devoting myself to being a mother. The plant spirits know and understand this. In fact, they have once again guided me to this awareness and next step. I am grateful for our friendship and trust where it leads. **Dr Lisa Lichtig, medical doctor, herbalist, and Mara'akame, USA**

I was lucky enough to study plant spirit medicine with Eliot which was a truly life changing experience. Not only did I learn a beautiful and effective form of healing, but I was also introduced to the healing power of fire through the Sacred Fire Community, and to a path of pilgrimage in the Huichol tradition. I honestly feel that my rosemary experience (described on p. 136) was the key to a doorway that has opened up a very different life, one that I could not have imagined possible for myself. Eliot introduced us to a very simple fire ceremony where we would make offerings to the fire to consecrate it. We learned that these were the Huichol (Wixarica) people's traditional offerings to Grandfather Fire (Tatewari) and that they helped us to connect with the divine energy of fire, our own hearts and path in life, and to each other. I felt so blessed to be able to attend these fires because I was painfully shy in those days, and found being in a group of people for a whole week at a time while studying PSM, very challenging and intense! It brought up all my fears beautifully and I found that being around a consecrated fire really helped me to quieten my mind. When an opportunity came up to train as a fire keeper I jumped at the chance. I have been holding monthly fires at my home now for the past twelve years which has been a very rewarding experience for myself and my community.

Sitting around these wonderful fires I would pray for help to find my path in life, because although I loved being a PSM healer I still felt like there was something else I was supposed to be doing. I just didn't know what it was. I began to have a series of very powerful dreams that had a very specific energy about them; they frightened me and I tried to ignore them, but I just couldn't forget them. In fact the energy of them seemed to intensify until I felt that I was going mad. It was at that point that I finally plucked up courage to tell Eliot. He explained that I was being called to pilgrimage to a specific site in

Mexico. As soon as he said this my heart knew it was right even if my mind was freaking out with fear! So began an incredibly mysterious, magical adventure to Mexico as an apprentice in the Wixarica tradition. I was initiated in 2017 after pilgrimaging to Mexico for seven years. My seemingly random experience with rosemary opened a doorway to a very surprising path, and I have a feeling the journey has only just begun. Thank you to rosemary, mugwort, and all the plants, Tatewari, the Wixarica people and last, but not least, Eliot Cowan for courageously paving the way for us all to follow in his steady, sure footsteps. **Anne Lynn, PSM healer, SFC fire keeper, and Mara'akame, UK**

My journey to becoming a Mara'akame (healer) in the Huichol tradition started with my relationship with plants. I was drawn to plant spirit medicine: it began with receiving the medicine which really helped me to open up to so many things, get in touch with my emotions and spirit for the first time in my life, find balance, and be open to learning in a new way. It was through the medicine of the plants that I was called to make pilgrimage and later be initiated as a Mara'akame. This also led me to work in service to my current way of life. Six years ago I became the executive director of the Blue Deer Center, which is a home for ageless wisdom and plant spirit medicine. We see the importance of reconnecting to the natural world around us and how we as human beings can remember our place in relationship with the world … it is where we find our balance and peace. "In the final embrace of gratitude, who can distinguish the giver from the receiver?" (inspired by Brother David Steindl Rast). **Mark Gionfriddo, Mara'akame and executive director of the Blue Deer Center, USA**

Not everyone has a calling to deep shamanism; it demands a high level of commitment underpinned by a specific spiritual alignment. And there are other paths of service. As we have said, the element of the heart is fire; fire makes the spark of attraction, from our own desires right through to the atomic level and the chemical foundation of life. We know that fire in its pure elemental form brings us warmth, light, connectedness, and wisdom. A project closely allied to plant spirit medicine is that of the Sacred Fire Community (SFC). Sacred fire provides opportunities for people to engage with fire and discover a path of personal and societal healing. We humans have had a relationship with fire for tens of thousands of years. Anthropologically, the first human use of fire is thought to have happened 800,000 years ago, and for the ancestors of our ancestors, opening this relationship was the defining spark in human awareness. Fire is the essence of heart—both individually and communally—holding our deepest knowing, wisdom, and the awakening connection to who we are, to each other, and to the greater world.

In these times of uncertainty and rapid change, it is common to feel increasingly disconnected from ourselves, each other, and the world. As the energy of transformation, fire is a primordial healing presence in all our lives. In the natural world, fire burns away deadwood and decay allowing forests to be reborn into lushness. Likewise, the human heart longs to burn away fear and worn-out patterns, allowing a fresh start to rebuild life-sustaining connections.

As a sacred fire fire keeper I (Lucy) have found that holding monthly community fires has enriched my life beyond measure. Around the fire together we sing, we laugh, we listen and hear about the challenges and joys that shape our lives. The role has also presented me with a host of challenges that have been pivotal for my personal development, has brought me into contact with a load of interesting people, and given me a very special relationship with fire itself for which I am extremely grateful. Feelings connected with fire are at once timeless and entirely of the moment. Sparks of deep memory are triggered by the flames of transformation and warmth. Sacred fire as simple medicine for human interaction has a place at all our hearths; it answers a profound longing in the most elemental way. The fire really is a very warm place.

The international Sacred Fire Community is led by elder Don David Wiley, who along with fire chief Annie King, supports the fire keepers with ongoing training. One extraordinary phenomenon that has manifested at this time is Grandfather Fire itself speaking to us directly;

> We have entered a period of great imbalance, where entire ecosystems, species, cultures and, perhaps soon, even humanity itself are being driven to the edge of extinction. When peoples in the past have come to such crisis points, their stories tell us that Grandfather Fire has appeared in a way that allows him to speak to the people, providing direct guidance and needed connection to the Divine.
>
> Similarly for our times, Grandfather Fire has made Don David into such a conduit, which the Huichols call an axihuatakame, or "spirit-speaking person". Under special ritual circumstances, Grandfather raises Don David's temperature to a high-fever

level, sending him into a coma-like state and enabling Grandfather to use his body to communicate with those in attendance. Although this phenomenon may seem strange to us, it is common to many of the original traditions of the world, such as the nechung oracle of Tibet, the heyoka of the Lakota, and the oracle of the ancient Greeks.

Several public Grandfather Fire audiences are held each year around the world. (From the website of Don David Wiley, www.keepsthefire.org)

Always, fire is guiding us to deepen our understanding of the heart-mind dilemma. This topic is deeply explored in *Heard Around the Fire*:

> The mind can be very talkative. It can worry, fret, obsess, plan and organise, all within a few seconds, day in and day out. Sifting through the chatter is a lot of work. You must learn the mind's voice and the heart's voice before you will know how to live from the heart. The heart has a direct connection to divine. (Jeff Baker, *Heard Around the Fire—Teachings of Grandfather Fire*, 2010)

Many who come to plant spirit medicine are touched by the fire—and vice versa. For some, sitting around a sacred fire ignites a calling and sparks the desire to become a fire keeper themselves.

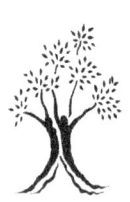

Soon after my return from the Pyrenees and my encounter with pokeweed, I came across the book *Plant Spirit Medicine* by Eliot Cowan. I read it and contacted the PO box and enrolled with his class in Massachusetts in 1999. I'd earned my living as a carpenter and joiner up until then so this was all very new to me and I was delighted by the whole experience. A new world opened to me, a world of wonderful possibilities. Along with a lot of technical stuff I learned a practical and simple technique to contact the spirit of plants.

Most of us in the class were boarding and quite often in the evening after supper we would gather in the tepee around the fire. I watched as people made offerings to the fire and walked around it—this put me outside my comfort zone. But there was a great man sitting there. Eliot I saw as a man who seemed to have lost his ego someplace. Over the years I grew to have a huge respect and love for him. Here at last was an authority I knew I could trust—what a relief! Over time my questions were answered by listening to Eliot's answers to others without me needing to speak. I became connected to the spirit of the fire and began to make the offerings myself. Whichever way you look at it the universe is an incredible dance of equilibrium and exchange. I saw the offerings as a gesture that recognised the gifts we get from the elemental fire.

At my home in Cornwall I made a fire-pit and invited people to come and sit around it and in 2005 I found myself in North Carolina training with another great man, very different from Eliot but of the same ilk as far as integrity and humour are concerned. I was taught by Don David Wiley how to become a fire keeper and was initiated by Grandfather Fire. We mostly speak about the fire in the male form, but without thinking about it when I light a fire I usually talk to it as she, as in "There she goes." I promised to keep a consecrated community fire, that is one to which offerings were made, every month for the rest of my life. Thirteen years and many fires later, this is my favourite job. **Michael Locke, plant spirit medicine healer and SFC fire keeper, UK**

I started going to monthly fires. I got introduced to Tatewari or Grandfather Fire, the spirit of the element of fire whose tradition comes from the Huichol people in north-west Mexico. I was drawn to the fires and realised I wasn't excited—it was a calling. It made so much sense to me. So I stood up, made myself accountable, applied myself. I went through a training which opened so many doors for me. In Mexico I received this initiation from a wonderful shaman called Don David Wiley, and I came back to Wales and continued. So now I have this relationship with the spirit of fire, I hold my own fires on a monthly basis. And this is down to circles within circles, it's a door that opened to me since I started receiving the medicine of the plant spirits. So now I can feel the natural world again, it's helping me just by holding these fires—my ego is diminishing, my confidence is growing, my relationship with spirit is growing, my understanding of the emotions and my patience and understanding with people who come to the fire are also growing. I'm being of service, I'm opening my home to people I don't really know—which I would have had problems doing before. I now welcome people in to receive the beautiful medicine of fire. I'm an initiated fire keeper with the Sacred Fire Community, a lifelong commitment which I'm so grateful to have made. Just like my relationship with the plants and Mother Nature. I now believe I'm a steward of this earth and I'm responsible for my being. I have a fantastic relationship with Grandfather Fire and who knows what door is next going to open for me! I'm now living and leading such a full life. It's beautiful. All thanks to plant spirit medicine. **Simon Earle Huxley, SFC fire keeper, Wales, UK**

Sitting by the fire the commitment to humanity, for life, spoke to me. It was something I was drawn to because it was so lovely. It makes me want to cry. Ahh! It's heart, it touches something. It's so simple and yet … It's like breath. You need your heart to be touched—I needed my heart to be touched. It touched my heart, and I thought it was important that it touched other people's hearts. Let the natural world of the element fire, Tatewari, Grandfather Fire come into your heart, bringing the excitement of creation and passion into your life whilst acknowledging sadness, fear, and loss. **Carole Nomessin, SFC fire keeper and PSM healer, UK**

Life is layered. Overlapping and tangled. Before one story ends another begins. So it is with the story I want to tell of how I became a fire keeper. It has many beginnings. It begins with a boy sitting beside a camp fire. My father was the warden at Kinver Scout Camp—a twenty-three-acre woodland. I grew up among those oaks and elms. From Monday to Friday I lived and went to school in a distinctly urban environment. But every weekend Dad released me into the woods where I met with other children of the Kinver Camp Guild. Together we built dens, climbed trees, broke bones, and forged lifelong bonds. Sometimes, the best times, we got to stay overnight and, then, we built campfires, gathered around them, and told each other stories. I always loved the fires. I always loved the stories. I recognised that something special happened in the light from the flames. There was magic here.

It begins lying on a treatment couch set up in my garden in the gentle warmth of a May afternoon. My back had gone into spasm again. It does so at regular intervals. By this point, I had tried numerous treatments for my persistent back problem: osteopaths, chiropractors, physiotherapists. None of them did much good. When my back went I would be laid up for days. My neighbour Lucy Wells offered me a PSM (hole in one) treatment. I was, I have to admit, sceptical. But I was also in considerable pain and desperate. So Lucy came and did her stuff which seemed to be minimal to the point of non-existent. It was pleasant enough lying in the warmth of the sun, but I couldn't see how it was going to do my back much good. Still, I liked Lucy and didn't want to upset a neighbour, so I did as she asked. She told me to take it easy for the rest of the day and to drink plenty of water. I smiled. They always tell you to drink lots of water. Lucy went home, I went to the kitchen to get a glass of water. My back felt no better. It was still painful to walk. But, as I went towards the kitchen, I felt a strong urge to lie down on the floor. The moment I lay down I felt a most remarkable sensation—as if all the vertebrae in my spine had collapsed, one by one, like a line of dominoes, realigning themselves into a new shape. Like a wave down my spine, all the bones spontaneously readjusted their position. My bent, twisted spasm back all at once became an upright, healthy, functioning spine. And all the pain had gone. I leapt up and ran down to Lucy's house—"What the hell did you do to me!"

These two beginnings became two threads that slowly but inexorably wove back and forth, gradually binding themselves together. Impressed as I was by the results of my first PSM treatment, I was open to further suggestions from Lucy. She told me about the guy who had taught her this stuff, gave me his book to read and recommended that I attend his five-day healing camp. Because by this time, I wasn't just dealing with a bad back. By this time, I had been diagnosed with Parkinson's disease and was looking at having to give up my job teaching. This was how I came to be sitting around a fire with Eliot Cowan, listening to him explain the importance of fire. And the importance of heart. Which is pretty much the same thing. It all made a lot of sense to me. It spoke to the heart of that small boy sitting around the campfire listening to stories. I realised that the heart of the small boy was still inside me so I decided to become a fire keeper. Luckily, Lucy, as well as being a PSM healer, is also a fire keeper. She was able to be my sponsor—to hold my hand and show me how to take the first steps on a lifelong journey. A commitment to hold monthly community fires—a safe space for people to gather and speak from the heart. She showed me how to make offerings, how to hold the space. And the plants wove their medicine through her teaching me.

During this time, I also went for treatments. There was a lot of emotional trauma that I had buried somewhere deep inside and carried around with me for thirty years. My refusal to deal with a past event meant that it had become my dark and hidden secret. I carried the weight of it around with me. I never spoke of it. And, in the silence, it grew heavier and heavier. But I became so accustomed to its weight that I accepted it as normal. The plants knew that my unspoken past was dragging me down and forced me to confront it. Plants and fire worked together to support me. I said words that had needed to be said for thirty years. Truths were finally heard. And a weight was lifted. These days, I have learned to trust the plants and the fire. For me, they work together. A powerful team that are helping me find my way to a place where I can live with an open heart. A better, truer place. It is an incredible journey. **Andy Jukes, SFC fire keeper in training, UK**

Because the plants know us in their deep unfathomable way and assist us in the wholesome unfolding of our lives, we don't have to try to work everything out for ourselves. Thinking we are in control, that we have to work everything out, worry through all the options and possible scenarios, is a habit of mind. Plant spirit medicine helps to bring us into our hearts, where we simply know. This is also the fundamental effect of coming to the fire.

> **Heart beat**
> *My heart opens and closes*
> *A fish struggling to breathe.*
> *Love is the medicine*
> *To chase coldness away.*
> *The opening hurts,*
> *A cracking open, a stretch.*
> *But the cold closing, a numbness,*
> *Hurts more.*
> *I am afraid to open.*

A howl of pain bursts out,
Illuminating some ancient lonely
Place I'd rather not see.
But staying closed, half-alive,
Numb, terrifies me more.
Every moment, I am praying to open
Let go, let go
I never understood what it means,
Let go, let go
What does it mean?
Let go, let go
How can I do it?
Let go, let go
Who will catch me?
Let go, let go
Can I really love?
Let go, let go
Am I loved?
Let go, let go
Is it safe, to be here?
Let go, let go
Is it safe, to be alive?
Let go, let go
What will happen if ...
Let go, let go
The mind asks constant questions
Let go, let go
The heart knows.

(Pip Waller, 2011)

Others have been called to work with the weather via an indigenous Mexican tradition. Some of these initiated weather workers (Graniceros) live and work in the UK. I (Lucy) have been privileged to become involved in a project working with our resident Graniceros. This is an account of one of our outings.

The snow had fallen heavily the evening before. On the day of our departure all was under the spell of the cold quiet blanket. As we drove south-west we caught up with a swirling blizzard and only just made it through to our night's lodgings before the road became impassable. We were on our way to the weather mountain on Dartmoor for the spring equinox ritual work. Waking to another snow covered morning I wasn't sure we would be able to reach our friends' home from where we would set out at first by car and then on foot. The roads up onto the moor were covered in deep drifts and impacted ice. It occurred to me so deeply, that morning, how serious it is, our connection to the weather. Weather work as I understand it is about building good, respectful relationships with the weather beings. This might sound curious to a Western ear. My friends are crowned weather workers in the Nuaha tradition of Mexico and have made a lifelong commitment to undertake to do this work on behalf of us all. They were called to this path by unusual experiences with the weather, particularly lightning. Many of us are not familiar with this level of personal sacrifice in our busy money-earning orientation and might be suspicious of such commitment, but having the privilege of friendship with them I feel a deep respect and gratitude for their work and am very glad to be involved. Strangely enough when we came to get the car out of its snowbound parking place, the sun had thawed enough of a path and the main roads were now clear, shiny wet tarmac. The way up onto the moor felt as if it melted before us and, carefully moving over occasional patches of ice and snow, we were able to arrive at our destination and meet up with the rest of the group. Our friends have been working for a number of years now, making pilgrimages to the weather mountain to offer thanks for the blessings the weather bestows upon us, without which we would not survive. Dartmoor in Devon is the place where the predominant south-westerly winds first meet the land and from there, the rest of the British weather patterns are determined.

The next day we were up before dawn to breakfast ahead of sunrise when we began our day long fast from food and drink. Leaving the house a short while later in the declining dark we walked down to the river to a place where the cars had been left to avoid early morning treacherous ice. The roads were passable enough with careful driving until we arrived at an iced up snowdrift. Sat upon it was a grounded car. Its driver was glad to see us approaching. He was on his way to work and had got marooned. We got out to help just as the sun rose over the horizon and lit up this most beautiful day. The moor could have been the moon or Mongolia. The snow sparkled as the morning sun blinked on, red and rosy, causing diamonds to appear on the wind sculpted drifts. Men got out shovels. And women?: we danced to the sun and its ability to move through even this fiercest display of winter.

It is the equinox, when light equalises with dark, the midpoint between two extremes. Two van loads of Romanian workers appeared coming up the road on their way to work; with their youthful strength they had no problem freeing the stranded car and they then seemed to disappear as quickly as they had come. We were free to continue and although the ice needed cautious driving we made it to the parking place from where we continued on foot. Dark clouds loomed away to the west as we trudged across a snow-laden moor. It wasn't easy terrain and deep drifts further hampered the path. Honouring the forces that bring the weather would have been familiar to our ancestors, who knew their dependence and better understood the reciprocal arrangements for showing respect and gratitude than we do today.

For me in those moments of crossing the moor, I felt it such a privilege to be included in this basically humble ritual that was engaged with the awesomely potent and powerful weather. And the sun came out to shine and the cold that we had feared proved bearable. If the journey was seriously strenuous it only seemed to create even more felt meaning and as we came down off the moor at last to return home, we found the roads completely clear. We drove back to the setting of the sun. The beauty of the celestial balancing act and the benevolence of the weather beings seemed to grace us with their magnificent acknowledgement.

The beauty and dedication of this path of service to the world and its weather is further described here by a crowned weather worker resident in the USA.

In 1989 my beloved teenage daughter abruptly passed away. For the year following I pretty much stayed close to the earth, somehow knowing this was the only thing that was going to get me through the loss. I was sleeping outside by the fire a lot, and walking every day. A number of plants would be calling to me, and I would be drawn to sit with them, and invariably I'd get messages and healing, being shown a bigger picture of my daughter's life and mine. There were a lot of messages from the trees, plants, and from the wind in the trees. I could hear something coming and soothing me, calming me. So at the end of that year, I heard my daughter's voice coming on the wind from the top of the trees, saying, "Don't be afraid to live your life without me," and that I had to get on with my life. That helped me to see that I wasn't really living my life. I was living, but not really fully in this world with my fellow human beings. In looking back over that year, I thought, "Wow, I received so much healing from these plants that called me to them over and over again. And if you can get that from a plant by sitting with them, what would it be like to learn how to make medicines and offer that to people, that healing?" So I set out to become a herbalist and for seven years I studied and practised herbalism.

At the end of those years, Eliot's book just fell into my lap. I was in a bookstore and it fell off the shelf and landed on me. I picked it up and started reading it and just started shaking … I thought, "Oh my god, this is what happened, it was the spirit of the plants that were healing me!" I didn't have to learn how to make medicines—though I was grateful I'd learned all of that. But immediately I knew my next step. I thought, "I've got to find this man, he's supposed to be my teacher." After meeting him and in talking with him, I immediately signed up for his classes.

The first time he taught us how to do a plant journey, which was to Artemisia. I went into this journey and the twin spirit of this plant showed itself to me, standing in front of a beautiful wind-shorn juniper type of shrubby tree. In conversing with it I asked it what I could give in return for the healing and medicine it was offering, and it told me to go to a local mountain and take an offering. I agreed very wholeheartedly and excitedly … then I came out of the journey and I thought, "Oh my gosh, what is an offering, and what mountain?!" I had no idea where I was supposed to go and what I was supposed to take.

For the offering, every spring I would put a small offering in my garden, for the plants and the earth and so on. This seemed right to take to the mountain. It became clear that the "local mountain" was a very sacred mountain near where I lived. I didn't know it was sacred at the time—actually I didn't even find that out until years later. It is a popular hikers' destination. So I climbed up to the top of the mountain with my small offering, with tons of other people. When I headed out it was an absolutely crystal clear blue sky, not a cloud in the sky, a gorgeous spring day. So I get up there and I'm looking around and think, "Where am I supposed to put this offering?" Well, out of the corner of my eye I see the shrubby tree from my plant journey. The tree that was behind the twin spirit of Artemisia, and it's wind-shorn because it's bare up there. There was a little rocky ledge behind this shrubby tree, and I thought, "Oh, I could go back there and no one would actually see me." So I went behind the tree and I start to say some prayers, and I'm in tears because I'm so grateful that I'm seeing this thing that I saw in the journey, you know, this is where I'm supposed to be!

I started to dig a little space with my hands for the offering I brought, and then I realised people are rushing past me. They're going down some of these trails, close to where I am. And I look up and there's a huge black cloud, perfectly round, that has come up over the mountain. It's coming straight towards me. People are clearing off the mountain because there could be lightning with no place to take cover. It scared me so bad! I knew I needed to get off this mountain! So I finished my prayers and offerings and jumped up and ran like the rest of the people. I was the last one to come down that trail, running down, feeling like the cloud was right over my shoulder, following me the whole way down the mountain. So I got down and the cloud had gone! It had moved on. It had completely disappeared. It was a completely clear day. Not a white cloud in the sky, much less a very ominous black cloud. I didn't say anything to Eliot in those years; probably if I had, "something else" would have happened ...

When I graduated from plant spirit medicine healer training, I did practise this beautiful medicine for three plus years, alongside my herbal practice. But then in 2002 my late husband became ill and I stopped my practice altogether. After his passing I began making pilgrimage to a sacred site with Eliot. It was in the first few years of pilgrimaging that this "something else" happened. I was asking the site, "What is my role, what is my service, what am I here for?" The weather beings showed up again. They showed up with so much force that I couldn't deny it any more. I had several warnings. The last warning was a blue orb coming out of a lightning storm from across the field, coming through a window in my house and right in front of my face! It was like a shot across the bow! I felt I had to say something before they struck again. I was directed to an elder shaman of the weather working Nahua tradition in the Central Highlands of Mexico. He performed a divination, and said, "This is a calling ... you are being called by the weather gods!"

In that moment I realised I'd always been connected to the weather. Growing up on the gulf coast of Texas, there were always tornadoes, hurricanes, wild winds, and storms. I actually loved it! I've always loved it. I've always loved being with the weather and a part of it. My mother had that connection too. When a hurricane was arriving, she always knew whether the family needed to leave or to ride it out at home. She always called it accurately and knew what to do.

When I received the divination of my calling, I was quickly discovering that my prayers at the pilgrimage site were being answered. Working with the weather beings is a major part of my soul, of who I am, of my service to the world. In 2006 the elder who had performed my divination initiated me as a weather worker, or Quiatlzques, in the tradition of the Nahua people. As a weather worker I help to keep alive for my people the ancient relationship of love and respect for those great sacred beings who provide the waters that all of us depend on for our lives to continue and prosper. Every year during our ceremonies we bring our offerings, our prayers and love on our altars in gratitude. And we experience that the weather responds with generosity to us, as those ancestors before us experienced for so many thousands of years.

In the past few years I have also been accepted onto the path of learning to perform the healings of this beautiful path. All of this feels natural, familial to me now, as if in rediscovering my family I have been rediscovering myself and my relationship to the divine. I am deeply grateful to my teacher for bringing me on this beautiful path of service, and to my teacher's teacher and to the long line of teachers before them. I will always be grateful to the plant spirits for bringing so much healing into my life. And after all these years, I still marvel at how the first plant spirit I met knew me so well and cared enough to patiently help me discover myself and my life's work. **Victoria Reeves, USA**

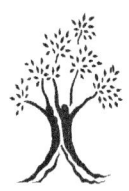

Involvement with plant spirits and time spent with fire has directed others to various pilgrimage paths. As the signature of heart-centred healing opens us to know what is demanded of us the hunger of the search and the unfolding of options appear with greater clarity. There is such value in discovering an authentic lineage to satisfy our yearning for a path with heart. One such lineage is that of the Egyptian goddess.

I sat alone by the fire in a tepee in a field in north Wales. The small space started to feel full of invisible beings but I wasn't afraid. As I watched the fire I felt ignited. I had a complete knowing that I should visit Mexico. One particularly special plant told me, "Go to the heart of the mother." I didn't know what this meant but it seemed connected. I was surrendering to guidance in the moment. It was exciting and scary, the love and guidance from the plants helping to hold me steady. I had also made contact with another woman, Diana, who I had been mysteriously told might have some information on the strong link I had been feeling with the deities of ancient Egypt and past life experiences there. I immediately recognised her as soon as I met her; I knew this was an old and strong soul connection. She told me that she had been tasked by spirit with the job of identifying people who were carrying soul fragments of a particular lineage. This lineage of women over many, many years and lifetimes had refined their capacity to embody the divine creative force of life. They were revered by the pharoahs with whom they held Egypt in a state of balance and harmony. As the ages turned, the lineage was destroyed, and the soul fragments of the lineage became more and more scattered. Now, as the Divine Feminine is returning, it is time for the lineage to heal and help to bring that divine energy back into the world.

The time in Mexico turned out to be one of profound healing, synchronicities unfolded one after another, I found the ideal house to rent, I received healing from a wonderful Mexican woman, Laura. I made friends, attended sacred fires, and received healing from a traditional Huichol healer. The heart of the mother in me was being nourished, but there was more ... part of the healing and re-empowering of the lineage was the opportunity to make a sacred pilgrimage to a sacred site of the Divine Mother. When the dates of the pilgrimage were announced the pilgrimage ended one day before my pre-booked flight home! I put my name down. I have attended eight pilgrimages up to date. It has been a profound journey to the heart of the mother, bringing challenges, deep healing, and reconnection with myself and everything and everyone around me. **Lynn-Amanda Brown, interspecies communicator, creative kinesiologist, and SFC fire keeper, Wales, UK**

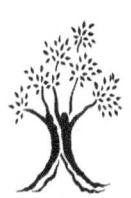

Whatever journey we take during our lifetime one certain thing is that at the end of this life we will die. Artist and gardener Jane Tibbotts was studying plant spirit medicine while living with aggressive cancer. She drew and wrote and gave her heart to her plant friends. Her partner describes the time leading up to her death.

Jane took Artemisia as a healing herb. She had it around too, it was quite special to her. She had a couple of dreams over a series of days, she tried to capture in the drawing. It was a bird, ascending up into the sky. The first picture was like an eagle and it had a heart around it. Then after a few more days she had another dream and the next picture it looked like a dove going up into the sun. She never understood the compelling message the plant was giving her.

The day that she died she gave me express instructions to phone a death doula to help her on her dying journey. The doula experienced that she and Jane went up high, through the celestial gates, to God's Chair, and at that point Jane changed her form into a dove—the emissary of peace. This is what was really important to her in her life. The Artemisia was the vehicle for helping her access that.

You can see the image Jane created from her plant dream on the back cover. Wherever your own journeys take you, we wish you the blessings of the plants and many rich and fruitful encounters. This quiet revolution wants to return us to truly being human. The plant spirits offer gentle yet far-reaching assistance for a purposeful way to live in alignment.

See the wind call attention to the trees
feel a sweetness coming to you on the breeze
divine nature, calling the way
wake up!

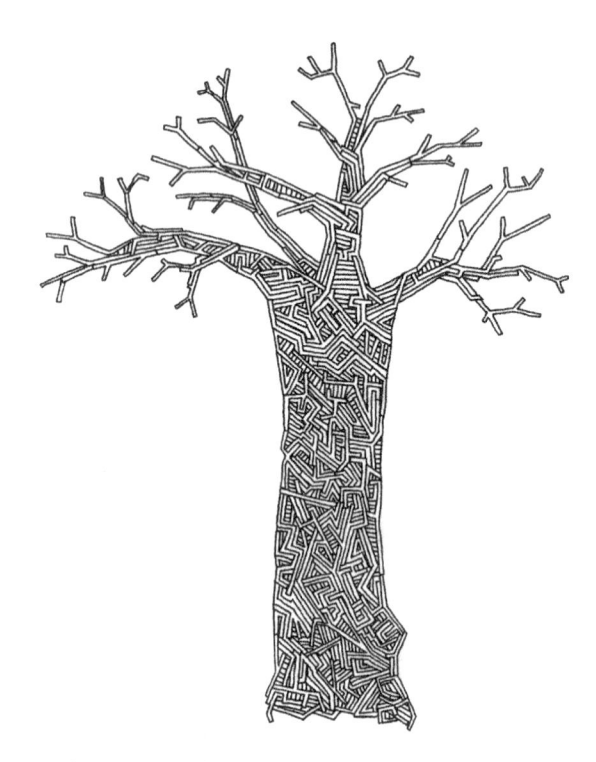

Geometric Tree by Asa Fusek Peters.

APPENDIX A — PLANT SPIRIT MEDICINE TODAY

Ever since the first publication of Eliot's seminal book *Plant Spirit Medicine* in 1995 so much has happened in the world of plant spirit and human relationships. After some years of practice Eliot began to teach the medicine to others, kindling great interest and helping many people reconnect to the long dormant approach of communicating with mutual respect between the human and plant kingdoms to access healing medicine. He regularly taught healer training courses in the States and has also taught in the UK, Canada, and Australia. With the growing number of PSM healers came a professional body, the PSMA, the Plant Spirit Medicine Association which supports the development of the medicine, presents annual conferences, and helps to ensure that healers are offering the medicine at the highest level of competence and skill possible. You can find those in Eliot's lineage who choose to join the PSMA on the website, www.plantspiritmedicine.org. You may find other healers who trained with Eliot (or elsewhere) who are also extremely dedicated and skilful, but as we are unable to vouch for these you would need to do your own exploration.

If you feel intrigued to learn more about the medicine, you might like to go to a talk or take a taster class to be introduced to plant spirit medicine in an experiential way. Many individual healers offer talks, workshops, and short courses. We offer introductory weekends fairly regularly in the UK, and have also taught in Switzerland and Germany. These courses are complete in themselves, aimed at encouraging deeper nature connection in participants and teaching what has come to be known as the shamanic or dream journey and plant study to connect directly with the spirits of plants. We are evolving ways of continuing and deepening study with those people who have attended our introductions to include seasonal work and the honouring of old cyclical festivals of the year. See our website www.touchedbynaturepsm.co.uk. If there is no course in your area and you want one, feel free to invite us.

We hope that many of you will be called to the path of becoming a dedicated plant spirit medicine healer, for the benefit of all our people. This is a message directly from Eliot Cowan for you:

> I hope this book is touching you in a new, yet familiar way. It could be that without even being aware of it, you have been longing to be touched this way. Plant spirits have a way to deliver a touch that puts us in a good way with our lives. I am convinced we all need such a sacred touch from time to time. There is great need for Plant Spirit Medicine, so we are preparing more healers to deliver this mysterious medicine. The world also needs more teachers to bring those who would be healers into the sacred dream of nature. Alison and I are working to guide people on the journey to becoming teachers of Plant Spirit Medicine.

The home of plant spirit medicine is in the USA at the Blue Deer Center (BDC) PO Box 905, Margaretville, NY 12455, in the Catskill Mountains. As the headquarters for plant spirit medicine it is also an important home for traditional teachings and practices of heart. Contact the center for information on plant spirit medicine and all aspects of the work of Eliot Cowan as well as the offerings of other traditional healers, teachers, and ceremonial leaders: www.bluedeer.org, telephone (001) 845 586 3225.

It is still possible to train directly with Eliot, who works with his senior teacher and PSM healer Alison Gayek. At present healer training courses are taught by Alison and Eliot in tandem. You can register your interest and find out more on the BDC website.

We conclude with this lovely piece which was generously contributed by Anna Murray-Preece, a PSM healer from Dartmoor. It expresses beautifully something about the wholeness of the practice of the medicine, so we offer it here in its entirety, although we have quoted some of it here and there in various chapters of this book.

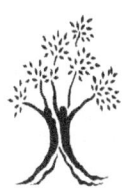

The Unfolding of our Remembering

A squeaking stops me. I have been walking quite quickly up the beautiful wooded valley, stepping from rock to rock and dodging fallen trees as I climb upwards on the soft mossy path. I am still now, taking in the chill, the damp atmosphere and lush green plants by the fast running stream. But who is it that is speaking? Two tall oaks rubbing bodies, their voices persistent and urgent call me.

Slender trunks, reaching to sunlight, silhouetted, dark and determined, softly cloaked in ivy and moss. They wave in a hypnotic, slow, gentle, rhythm as the wind catches their branches, stilling my mind and opening my senses.

I hear the rushing burble of the stream and the ever changing breath of the wind. I see clouds dance through the clear blue sky.

I feel the breeze gently licking my body and cooling the skin on my face.

Birds caw and twitter, my breath rises, then falls as it enters and leaves my body.

Feet firmly on the ground I find myself responding to the waving trees. As I sway back and forth the wind blows stronger as if to say "Hello" as it often does when I honour its presence.

I am dropping into the dream of nature.

My heart softens and expands; I become increasingly aware of being part of this. I am the trees, I am the stream, I am the river, I am the earth, and I am also myself. I am aware of the familiar feeling of subtle, blissful, light energy that comes when I give a plant spirit medicine treatment.

Entering the "dream of nature" seems to be for some, one of the "side effects" of practising or receiving plant spirit medicine. My clients often come back after a treatment reporting a heightened awareness of nature. Layla describes this beautifully:

> Plant Spirit Medicine has profoundly changed my life. I spent years with very little self-love, feeling lost and suffering the effects of past trauma. I felt the result of this amazing healing almost immediately. It started to give me the confidence to be who I am authentically. I started to let some things go; friendships, job, diet etc. that weren't serving me positively, and at the same time pull positive things towards me; friendships, life decisions etc. I started to face up to old hurts and trauma and work through them, incredibly hard at times, but necessary. I recovered from an autoimmune disease. Every time I have a treatment I seem to go deeper into this amazing healing with the plant spirit that my practitioner (Anna) has chosen for me. It's deeply physically relaxing and brings incredible clarity and groundedness.
>
> My last treatment was mind blowing, I felt completely connected to all of nature. I felt the plant spirits calling me. It suddenly felt as if I'd wandered into a dream. I have never seen nature in this way before ... I came across a frosty field; it was glistening, magical, crystal-like, completely breathtaking. I think the plant spirits had given me a glimpse into their world.
>
> I'm so grateful for everything Anna has done for me, but when I tell her this, she very humbly replies "But it's not me, it's the plant spirits."

I almost asked her to take that last bit out because as soon as I read it I realised both the truth and the folly in my response and in not receiving her appreciation. It is of course from the plants that the healing comes, but the plant spirit medicine healer doesn't just sit back and observe. What I love about it is the collaboration that happens between myself, the client, the Chinese five elements diagnosis, and the plants.

The five elements bring our awareness to the rhythms and qualities of each of the seasons, each corresponding to an emotion. The wood element, for example, relates to the spring when the land awakens and the upward rising energy is so strong that we can almost see plants grow. Suddenly we are surrounded with colour, flowers, green, and leaves, so clearly reflected in the times when we feel energy and drive or an upward rising of anger. In autumn, the metal element, the falling leaves teach us how to let go when we grieve a loss or move from one phase of our life onto the next.

For me as a PSM healer, it is a continual process of learning how to be with and embody each of the qualities of the elements. How am I with anger, or with joy, how do I receive nourishment and then let go of things when they are finished? Am I able to rest at the end of it all? I need to be open to touch these places of ease and of discomfort. I am challenged to know myself better so that I may meet my clients in their elemental nature. This inner relationship also opens me to the plants and the natural cycles of the world we live in.

Recently, with small groups of people, I have been exploring the plants and the elements through an embodied awareness of each season. It has been fascinating to see how for some the spring is a time of excitement and new beginnings, their body is energised and ready for action. Then for others there is a feeling of sluggishness or resistance and a wish to stay resting in the stillness, the safe haven of winter. I was interested to see how the falling energy of autumn is reflected in people's body and movement, how for many it supported a letting go of old habits and more trust in the unknown.

It's late February and I am in the woods again. I lie on a soft bed of leaves my head resting on a mossy rock. As I look up, as before, the long, tall oaks gently wave from above and as I watch transfixed; gradually my capacity to listen, see, and feel opens. I love how each tree lightly brushes the edge of the other, meeting but giving space, touching then parting. My body responds, softly rocking on my lower back, my spine finding satisfying twists that echo the shape of the branches. I find my legs dancing with the sway of the trees. I am almost upside down, legs in the air, comfortable, as I nestle in my bed of leaves. In this position I begin to see, feel, and receive the woodland, the river, the sounds, and sensations more acutely. The sunlight lightly touches me, moving slowly downwards with the passing of time and with this I become aware of a sharp chill. My fingers become colder till in the end it is unbearable and in this season of winter, the water element, the cold reminds me of the need to survive, the knowledge that I am human and need heat and warmth. So then I walk, beside the rushing, bubbling, splashing, and diving of the delicious River Dart.

This opening to the senses that I experience when I enter the "dream of nature" is also integral to being a PSM healer. We need to listen to the sounds of our clients, to see them clearly, even to smell them! Through the sense of touch, we feel the pulses in order to diagnose changes in their response to the plants. I find that the more I am in relationship to my body, the ground, and my heart, the more my mind stops its chatter, its need to get it "right", and the more I can be present with and receive the other person in all his or her fullness.

What we call the "dream of nature" will touch each of us in different ways. For me it is a place of quiet, subtle awareness, where my perceptions are simultaneously heightened and yet softer. It relates to what in Buddhism is known as Sambhogakaya, the realm of our reality where we are opened to subtle energy, to dream, symbol, image, and feeling. This is where things are more fluid and where what has become stuck in us can move, heal, and transform.

Everyone responds to plant spirit medicine differently. Briony, for example, has a long-standing connection with the "little people" whom she has seen since childhood. Through this she is able to see and feel the plant spirits working on her: they "tugged and hauled at something long and sinewy which emerged from my finger", helping to heal her painful shoulder, which you read about in the piece on p. 52. Layla felt the benefits of PSM immediately, but her experience of being "called by the plants" happened more recently after many years of regular treatments. It is my experience that over time my awareness is increasingly opened to the rhythms and cycles of nature and the subtlety of plant energies. Each of us is attuned to plant spirit medicine in our own way. For some changes happen very gradually and it is only over time that the depth of healing becomes clear. For others the healing is signified by a change in perception. Rob says: "During the course of a session I may notice a clarifying of my awareness, my vision clears, a bit like mist clearing, it is then only gradually that I have a sense of how my whole system is changing and my underlying sense of well-being returns; it can be a few hours later when I begin to feel physical symptoms shift."

I think, however, that most people experience the gentle nudge of the plants and a sense of returning to a more heart centred awareness. For me there is often a very clear feeling of being "in balance". I have the good fortune of having had treatments from Lucy while teaching meditation and movement retreats. This meant that my sensitivity to the changes I was experiencing was heightened. I could feel the energy in my body shift and open. My meditation could go deeper and stiller and my body felt more fluid and relaxed. From this came physical changes, as my menopausal hot flushes reduced and my sleep deepened.

My relationship to the world is in general very kinaesthetic. When I do a journey to a plant I often feel a lot of sensation in my body. One example of this is in relation to a fire plant that I work with. In my dream journey, I experienced a lot of joy and pleasure, which relates to the fire element. The plant spirit anointed and massaged my body, followed by a swim in a bubbling jacuzzi-like part of the river. Whenever I give this plant medicine, I re-enter this dream and the joy of the journey. Another plant took me through the petals of its flower to the portal between birth and death, a profound opening that I feel through my whole body when I administer this plant to a client. Another plant has the effect of my heart feeling soft and open each time I think of it, while another gives me the feeling of the holding of a loving community, helping me to feel a sense of belonging. One of my plants took me to a high ledge above a huge expanse where I find myself able to feel the awe of this without the terror. As someone who is afraid of heights this is an especially wonderful experience.

The generosity of the plants continually amazes me. In exchange for the simple offering of oat groats that I give before a plant journey, they give so much healing and seem so happy that we are reunited with them.

I have called this piece The Unfolding of our Remembering, because I feel that what PSM does is to enable each of us, healer and client, to begin to remember what is innate in us. This is the memory of our deep relationship and interconnectedness with nature, the plants, and all its elements. Through this we are gradually invited closer to our heart and into the dream of nature.

Anna Murray Preece, PSM healer and psychotherapist, UK (with excerpts from Layla, Briony, and Rob)

APPENDIX B — ACORN MAGIC

To make acorns fit for eating, the tannic acids need to be washed out. There are two ways to do this—one is by using running cold water, the other by boiling and repeatedly replenishing the water with fresh.

You dry them indoors for a couple of days, then shell and put them into a net or sock, tying it securely in a river or stream for 3–5 days. Alternatively you can boil the shelled acorns in a large amount of water. Every hour you discard the water and replace with fresh three times. After that, taste an acorn and if it is still bitter, boil them again. When they are no longer bitter, mash them and let cool a little. Strain through a strainer lined with cloth; gather the cloth and squeeze as much water out as possible. Then spread the mush out on the cloth somewhere warm to dry. This usually takes at least 2 days. Put in a dehumidifier to speed up the process. Grind it to flour in the coffee grinder and store in a jar. If totally dry it will keep 6–12 months.

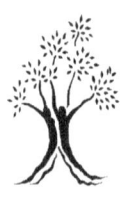

Acorn cookies

Ingredients: 1 cup butter or margarine
¾ cup honey (or 1 cup brown sugar)
About 3½ cups acorn flour (opposite)
1 generous cup all-purpose flour
1 teaspoon baking powder

To make: Preheat the oven to 350°F. Melt the butter and honey, then add the other ingredients. Stir and let cool until the dough stiffens up enough to roll into balls (golf ball size or smaller). Place the balls on a greased baking sheet and press down into flat cookie shapes. Bake in the oven for 10–15 minutes, until golden brown. Transfer to a wire rack to cool. Makes about 30 cookies. Keeps 10–14 days in an airtight container.

This recipe was given by PSM healer Anna Richardson, and first published in *The Herbal Handbook for Home and Health* (Pip Waller, 2015).

CONTRIBUTORS

Buffy Aakaash, PSM healer and SFC Firekeeper. Buffy is a healer, poet, playwright, chef, and business owner living in western New Mexico, in an area known as "Ancient Way". As a Firekeeper with Sacred Fire Community, he helps to train others to hold space for community fires around the world. He sends gratitude to the plants and all of Nature for giving him his life.
aakaash3404@gmail.com www.buffyspiritmedicine.com
www.buffyaakaashcompany.weebly.com

Laura Leonor Sanchez Andrade, PSM healer and massage & bodywork therapist, Mexico. Laura lives and practises in Amatlan de Quetzalcoatl, Tepoztlan, Mexico. In addition to being a plant spirit medicine healer, Laura is qualified in acupressure massage, Gestalt therapy, bio-energetic therapy, reiki, and polarity. She is also a teacher of yoga and acu-yoga and offers janzu (therapeutic meditation and relaxation in water).
0052 739 3933429 0052 777 4421794 email copalixchel56@hotmail.com

Kate Barrier, PSM healer and SFC fire keeper, USA. Kate Barrier began studying plant spirit medicine with Eliot Cowan in 2007. She holds a

degree in psychology and religion and a master's degree in education. She is a certified massage therapist and became an initiated fire keeper in the Sacred Fire tradition in 2014 and was identified as part of the Egyptian Goddess Lineage in 2015. Most recently she has served as the centre director for the Blue Deer Center in Margaretville, New York where she was mentored by a local Catskills beekeeper. Kate has made her home for the last 30 years in Michigan, USA where she stewards a parcel of land rich with native plants and trees.
katebarrier@aol.com

Louise Berliner, USA. Louise Berliner plays with words, herbs, fibre, and vine. She has a studio at the Umbrella in Concord, MA. Her poems, articles and short fiction have appeared in *VQR, The Mom Egg, Porter Gulch Review, Ibbetson Review, Sacred Fire* magazine, and plein air chapbook collections from Old Frog Pond and Fruitlands. She is the author of *Texas Guinan, Queen of the Night Clubs*, and when she isn't writing or weaving can be found walking at Great Meadows Wildlife Refuge. Artnspirit@verizon.net 001 978-318-0707

K'Anna Burton, PSM healer and SFC fire keeper, USA. K'Anna Burton lives in Michigan, USA. She has been involved in holistic healthcare, therapeutic bodywork and healing work for over twenty-five years. Her approach to life and healing is heart-centred and spiritually focused. K'Anna and her partner hold monthly community fires in Okemos, MI. kannaburton@aol.com

Lynn-Amanda Brown, interspecies communicator, creative kinesiologist and SFC fire keeper, Wales, UK. Lynn-Amanda lives in Snowdonia, north Wales, treating her two- and four-legged patients in her home and around the world via Skype. She holds monthly fire circles. www.lynn-amanda.com lynn-amanda@hotmail.co.uk

Rachel Corby, medicine woman and rewilding coach, UK. Rachel Corby trained with native plant spirit healers in Africa and South America. She completed the plant spirit medicine practitioner training with Eliot Cowan and a sacred plant medicine apprenticeship with Stephen Harrod Buhner. She is the author of three books; the most recent is *Rewild Yourself: Becoming Nature*. Rachel shares plant spirit connection

and rewilding through workshops, retreats, apprenticeships, and individual mentoring.
twitter/Facebook/instagram: @mugwortdreamer www.wildgaiansoul.com

Eliot Cowan, founder healer of PSM and tsauririkame (traditional elder healer in the Huichol tradition), USA. Eliot Cowan authored the book, *Plant Spirit Medicine*. He has been teaching, leading healing retreats, and maintaining a private practice for many years. He began to study and practise herbalism in 1969, then temporarily set it aside to study acupuncture. He received his licentiate, bachelor and master of acupuncture degrees from the late J. R. Worsley at the College of Traditional Acupuncture, Leamington Spa, England, and served on the faculty of that institution in 1979–1980. In the early 1980s, Eliot once again turned his attention to herbal healing. Following a recommendation by Dr Worsley, he began seeking the guidance of the plants themselves to support the healing of his clients. In this way, Eliot rediscovered the ancient shamanic practice of plant spirit medicine. Eliot has continued his healing work through the traditions of the Huichol people of Mexico. He completed his shamanic apprenticeship with the late Don Guadalupe Gonzalez Rios. www.bluedeer.org

Louisa Dix, PSM healer, UK. Louisa Dix BSc, MA, dipSW is a new traveller, living in and around the UK in the most low impact, off grid sustainable way she can manage. She is training in plant spirit medicine and is passionate about food as a medicine and natural healing.
qiunaverse@gmail.com

Michael Dunning, Yew Shaman, USA. During the late 1980s Michael became extremely ill as a result of an encounter in the far north of Scotland with an otherworldly being that he refers to as the Sulfur Daemon. Several years later and close to death, he was led to an ancient female yew tree in the south of Scotland. Michael spent over nine years under this yew where he was healed and given the template for a spiritual teaching and shamanic practice named the Yew Mysteries. Michael teaches the Yew Mysteries in the UK and the USA. He is currently writing a book about his experiences.
www.yewmysteries.com

Zoe Ekin, PSM healer, UK. Zoe is a mother of four beautiful children, wife, biodynamic smallholder, plant spirit medicine healer, and herbalist in training. She lives in rural Somerset.
zoe.ekin@gmail.com

Alison Gayek, PSM healer and senior teacher of PSM, USA. Alison Gayek lives in North Carolina where she has a plant spirit medicine practice. She also teaches plant spirit medicine. Courses include the plant spirit medicine healer training course, all manner of plant spirit medicine introductory classes and workshops, as well as continuing education courses for the PSM healers.
plantspiritsheal@gmail.com

Monika Ghent, PSM healer and herbalist, Canada. Monika is a plant spirit medicine healer and herbalist in Ontario, Canada. She also has a school of herbalism, Living Earth School of Herbalism, with her husband, Michael Vertolli, which offers general interest workshops and online classes, and certificate and diploma programmes in Western herbalism and related fields of study.
www.dreamingwillow.ca info@dreamingwillow.ca
www.livingearthschool.ca monika@livingearthschool.ca

Mark Gionfriddo, Mara'akame and executive director of the Blue Deer Centre, USA. A mara'akame (shaman) in the Huichol tradition and a granicero (weather shaman) in the Nahua tradition, Mark Gionfriddo began his Huichol shamanic apprenticeship training in 2003 under tsaurririkame Eliot Cowan of Santa Barbara, California. He was initiated as a granicero by Don Lucio in 2002.
markgionfriddo@bluedeer.org

Lucy Harmer, PSM healer, feng shui and space clearing expert, Switzerland. Lucy Harmer is a feng shui and space clearing expert, PSM healer, and an international author and teacher whose books include *Discovering Your Spirit Animal and Shamanic Astrology: Understanding Your Spirit Animal Sign*. Lucy is also founder and director of the Innerelf Centre, a thriving business that promotes transformative and inspirational living. Lucy is currently based in Sion, Switzerland.
www.lucyharmer.com

Rachel Tara Hargrave, PSM healer, drummer, and artist, Wales, UK. Rachel Tara Hargrave lives in west Wales where she has a plant spirit medicine practice and runs community drumming workshops. rhmojas@hotmail.com

Fiona Heckels and Karen Lawton, are Seed Sistas, Sensory herbalists and hopeful activists, UK. Karen Lawton and Fiona Heckels are advocates for the plants through initiating medicine gardens, writing and teaching about magical herbalism and grass roots growing. Their mission: to connect people with their local plants promoting empowerment, autonomy, freedom, and diversity in health care. They do this by facilitating grassroots growing projects and sharing their knowledge and passion about plant medicine to all who will listen!, believing that through community cohesion and reconnection to the Earth, positive change will ensue. www.sensorysolutions.co.uk

Nathaniel Hughes, herbalist and founder of the School of Intuitive Herbalism, UK. Nathaniel Hughes lives in Stroud and has developed a style of practice in herbalism weaving together somatic exploration, trauma integration, and working with plants as teachers and guides. He founded the School of Intuitive Herbalism where deep connection to the plants forms the core of training, and loves exploring the infinite lands of plant consciousness with his students. www.intuitiveherbalism.org.uk

Simon Earle Huxley, SFC fire keeper, UK. Simon lives in north Wales where he holds monthly community sacred fires. www.sacredfirecommunity.org

Sarah Hyde, naturopath and PSM healer, Wales, UK. Sarah Hyde lives on a smallholding in west Wales. She practises naturopathy and craniosacral balancing. She also teaches non-stylised movement and meditation, primarily in the landscape, to promote self healing, creativity, and reconnection to the elemental world.
sarahlhyde@yahoo.co.uk www.llandeilonaturalhealthcentre.co.uk

Barbara Jones, holistic vet, UK. Practising as a conventional vet since 1979, Barbara started to use homeopathy in her practice in 1985,

acupuncture in 1994, and then introduced more therapies as years went by. Out of deep concern for environmental sustainability, and the potential damage that can be caused to patients by inappropriate use of conventional medicines, she now practises mostly holistic therapies, including homeopathy, acupuncture, Western and Chinese herbs, reiki, flower essences, nutrition and plant spirit medicine.
www.vetholistic.co.uk

Andy Jukes, SFC fire keeper in training, UK. Andy Jukes lives in south Shropshire. He used to work in education but was forced to retire. He has Parkinson's disease. He walks his dog. He practises tai chi. Every month he holds a community fire. He writes a blog that documents the results of living within this condition.
andyjukes.wordpress.com

Jo Jukes, shiatsu practitioner (MRSS), artist, and creative therapist, UK. Jo Jukes is a registered shiatsu practitioner, teacher, artist, and creative therapist. Originally from Sheffield she has made Shropshire her home for the last twenty-five years and draws on nature and the landscape for her inspiration in all things.
jojukes.wordpress.com

Becky Knight, textile artist and teacher, Wales, UK. Becky is a textile artist and community arts facilitator based near Aberystwyth on the coast of mid Wales.
www.beckyknight.co.uk

Loredana Kraushaar, PSM healer, UK. Loredana came to PSM through a friend in 2006 and started training as a healer two years later. PSM has helped her rekindle her deep relationship to the natural world that continues to nurture and sustain her. She found relief from endometriosis and various digestive issues. She lives with her son and partner in Bristol where she shares a treatment room with a fellow practitioner.
loredana.psm@gmx.co.uk FB: Walking with beauty

Gemma Leighton, PSM healer and musician, UK. Gemma is a musician and PSM healer. She lives in Huddersfield.
www.gemm.band

Lisa Lichtig, MD and Mara'akame, USA. A devoted and heartful holistic family doctor, midwife, mother, and healer for over twenty years, Lisa further serves her greater community as a traditional healer and ceremonial leader.
www.familytofamily.org or lisa@familytofamily.org

Michael Locke, plant spirit medicine healer and SFC fire keeper, UK. Michael offers plant spirit medicine healing and monthly community fires. A master carpenter who loves to forage for food, medicines, wood, and anything, he is a lifelong devotee of Prem Rawat.
07936 638329 mjlocke@hotmail.com

Anne Lynn, PSM healer, SFC fire keeper and Mara'akame, UK. Anne Lynn lives in East Sussex where she has a plant spirit nedicine healing practice and holds a community fire and a women's fire every month.
kestrelswing@yahoo.ca

Jonathan Merritt, SFC fire keeper, Mara'akame, and poet, USA. Jonathan is a Mara'akame—an initiated traditional shamanic healer in the lineage of the Huichol people of Mexico—and a fire keeper for the Sacred Fire Community. He lives in Portland, Oregon, USA with his wife, the naturopathic physician Jennifer Means, and their two children, Maya and Eli. He is also the father of the actress/activist Madeline Merritt.
jonathan.l.merritt@outlook.com

Anna Murray Preece, PSM healer and psychotherapist, UK. Anna Murray Preece lives on Dartmoor and practises plant spirit medicine, rhythmic healing, and psychotherapy. She facilitates both Buddhist and nature based meditation and movement retreats. Her "Opening to Your Wild Body" seasonal weekends focus on attuning to our inner rhythm in relation to the rhythm of nature and the land.
http://www.healingfromthesource.co.uk
annamurraypreece@gmail.com

Peter Neumann, herbalist, candle and incense maker, and PSM healer, UK. Peter lives in Totnes. He has been making amazing candles and incense since 1983, and is the proprietor of Touchfire Candles. He has been a medical herbalist since 2002. He is training to be a PSM healer.
01803 849040 office@touchfire.co.uk

CONTRIBUTORS

Carole Nomessin, PSM healer, SFC fire keeper, UK. As an elemental medicine woman Carole incorporates elements from all her training and experience which included five elements acupuncture as well as many other healing techniques. Plant spirit medicine is at the core of who she is and within her work, and has given her great pleasure in her life and work. She is very grateful to Elliot Cowan, founder of Plant Spirit Medicine. Carole works with individuals, groups, and businesses. She is also a fire keeper.
0044 7727 188630 www.sacredfire.community nomessin@hotmail.com
FB: Elemental Medicine Woman

Annette Ramsay, Wales, UK, is a herbalist and artist, landscape gardener, biophiliac, and general lover of all things natural and green.
herbyfairy@yahoo.co.uk

Dawn Rafferty, PSM healer and writer, Ireland. Dawn Rafferty has been practising plant spirit medicine in Galway, West of Ireland since 2007. At the time of going to print, she is within the process of completing the requirements necessary to practise distance healing. Dawn is also a writer of the wisdom still alive and thriving in the land, plants, and elements.
dawn@earthlings.ie

Victoria Reeves, USA. Victoria Reeves is a mother, grandmother, wife, healer, and weather worker in the Nahua tradition living with her husband in the Catskill Mountains of New York.

Anna Richardson, PSM healer and forest school leader, UK. Anna works for Cultivating Curiosity as a forest school leader with children of all ages and with Circle of Life Rediscovery, training forest school leaders. She runs independent workshops on foraging and "Seeing through Native Eyes". She qualified in PSM in 2011 and also applies this training to her work with groups, helping people to connect with the plants and the natural world. She is a writer, her first book being *Learning with Nature: A How-to Guide to Inspiring Children through Outdoor Games and Activities* (written with Marina Rob and Victoria Mew).
www.circleofliferediscovery.com/index.php?page=anna-richardson

CONTRIBUTORS

Emyr Roberts, PSM healer, Wales, UK. Emyr Roberts lives in Waunfawr, Gwynedd with Lynn Amanda Brown, is father to Sara, and works as finance manager for Snowdonia National Park Authority.
emyrroberts@gmail.com

Phil Roberts, PSM healer and SFC fire keeper, Australia. Phil Roberts is a plant spirit medicine healer and fire keeper who lives in Perth, Western Australia.
www.philrobertspsm.com.au phil@philrobertspsm.com.au

Bex Syrett, UK, lives on the Welsh border, on the side of a limestone hill. She is fortunate to have land owned by the wildlife trust next to her own. She writes: "The hill is covered in wildflowers and native trees. We have rare butterflies, insects, and plenty of wildlife around us. I feel blessed."

Jane Tibbotts was a passionate lover of plants and a fine artist and writer. A botanist, gardener and nature lover, she began to study to be a plant spirit medicine healer in the last stages of a serious illness. She loved plant spirit medicine and said that being on the course was the highlight of her life at that time. Sadly, she died before the end of the course, from which her class-mates graduated in December 2018.

Michael Vertolli, herbalist, Canada. Michael Vertolli is a Western traditional herbalist practising near Toronto, Canada. He practises a system of herbalism that integrates a modern physiological approach with traditional wisdom based on a deep engagement with the world and the plant spirits. He is the director of Living Earth School of Herbalism.
www.livingearthschool.ca michaelvertolli.blogspot.ca

Julie Wood, PSM healer and herbalist, UK. Julie Wood lives near Shaftesbury, Dorset and completes her PSM training in December 2018. She works for Neal's Yard Remedies on its helpline, teaching herbal medicine, and has contributed to NYR books. She is also working with the Rewilding with the Labyrinth project, teaching deeper communication with spirit and the wild.
www.ladycomfrey.co.uk

ILLUSTRATORS

We would like to thank the artists for their generosity for allowing us to reproduce their work in this book. Here they are in order of appearance.

Touch Me Oak
Sarah Woolfenden
www.sarahwoolfenden.co.uk

Haemoglobin/Chlorophyll
Lucy Wells

Plant/animal cell
Lucy Wells

Woodland Scene
Jane Tibbotts

Mugwort
Parkinson's Herbarium

Lungwort
Rachel Lloyd
rachellloyd@hotmail.com
(Also thanks for the 'tree people' motif found throughout the book)

Winter Tree
Ian Collett
www.iancollett.wordpress.com

Comfrey
Michael Locke
(Also thanks for the 'herb robert' motif found throughout)

Elderflower
Pip Waller

Foxgloves
Rose Perry
roseperry01@gmail.com

Motherwort
Parkinson's Herbarium

Elecampane
Pip Waller

Hellebore
Lily Tonkin Wells
lilbobaggins@hotmail.co.uk

Geometric Tree
Asa Fusek Peters
asapeterss@gmail.com

Mugwort Journey – To the Light (back cover)
Jane Tibbotts

RESOURCES

Books

Baker, J. (2010). *Heard Around the Fire—Teachings of Grandfather Fire*. San Francisco, CA: Sacred Fire Press.

Brooke, E. (1992). *A Woman's Book of Herbs: A Witches Guide to Healing Body, Mind and Spirit*. London: The Women's Press [new indexed edition, 2107].

Buhner, S. H. (2002). *The Lost Language of Plants. The Ecological Importance of Plant Medicines to Life on Earth*. White River Junction, VT: Chelsea Green.

Cowan, E. (2014). *Plant Spirit Medicine*. Louisville, CO: Sounds True. (Rewrite of original *Plant Spirit Medicine*, 1995.)

Gawande, A. (2014). *Being Mortal: Medicine and What Matters in the End*. New York: Metropolitan Books.

Harner, M. (1980). *The Way of the Shaman*. San Francisco, CA: HarperSanFrancisco.

King, T. (1990). *All My Relations: An Anthology of Contemporary Canadian Native Fiction*. Toronto, Canada: McClelland & Stewart. Macfarlane, R., & Morris, J. (2017). *The Lost Words*. London: Hamish Hamilton.

McCraty, R. (2015). *The Science of the Heart*, Volume 2. San Jose, CA: The HeartMath Institute. http://store.heartmath.org/Science-of-the-Heart-Volume-2/science-of-the-heart.html

Nerburn, K. (2009). *The Wolf at Twilight, An Indian Elder's Journey Through a Land of Ghosts and Shadows*. Novato, CA: New World Library.

Prechtel, M. (2011). *An Unlikely Peace in Cuchumaquic*. Berkeley, CA: North Atlantic Books.

Robb, M., Mew, V., & Richardson, A. (2015). *Learning with Nature: A How-to Guide to Inspiring Children through Outdoor Games and Activities*. Green Books. https://www.amazon.co.uk/Learning-Nature-How-Inspiring-Activities/dp/0857842390

Turnbull, C. M. (1961). *The Forest People*. New York: Simon & Schuster.

Wall Kimmerer, R. (2015). *Braiding Sweetgrass: Indigenous Wisdom, Scientific Knowledge and the Teachings of Plants*. (Minneapolis, MN: Milkweed Editions.

Waller, P. (2015). *The Herbal Handbook for Home and Health: 501 Recipes for Healthy Living, Green Cleaning, and Natural Beauty*. Berkeley, CA: North Atlantic Books.

Waller, P. (2018a). *The Health and Beauty Botanical Handbook*—a shorter version of *The Herbal Handbook for Home and Health* with over 350 recipes. Brighton: Leaping Hare Press. https://www.quartoknows.com/Leaping-Hare-Press

Waller, P. (2018b). *Deeply Holistic: A Guide to Intuitive Self-care*. Berkeley, CA: North Atlantic Books.

Wohlleben, P. (2017). *The Hidden Life of Trees—What They Feel, How They Communicate: Discoveries from a Secret World*. London: HarperCollins.

Wood, M. (1997). *The Book of Herbal Wisdom: Using Plants as Medicine*. Berkeley, CA: North Atlantic Books.

Articles

Bassett, D., Tsosie, U., & Nannauck, S. (2012). Our culture is medicine: Perspectives of Native healers on posttrauma recovery among American Indian and Alaska Native patients. *Permanente Journal*, 16(1):19–27.

Matsuwa, Don Jose, Huichol, (1989). www.indigenouspeople.net/huichol.htm

Myers, Natasha. *Exploring Goethean Science*. www.schumachercollege.org.uk/learning-resources/exploring-goethean-science

Walker, G. H. (2016). Rediscovering what has always been there. www.indigenouspeople.net/under.htm

Richardson, M., Cormack, A., McRobert, L., & Underhill, R. (2016). 30 days wild: Development and evaluation of a large-scale nature engagement campaign to improve well-being. *PLOS ONE*, 11(2): e0149777. https://doi.org/10.1371/journal.pone.0149777

Useful websites

www.bluedeer.org
www.heartmath.org
www.keepsthefire.org
www.pipwaller.co.uk
www.plantspiritmedicine.org (to find a psm healer)
www.sacredfire.community
www.sacredfire.foundation
www.touchedbynaturepsm.co.uk

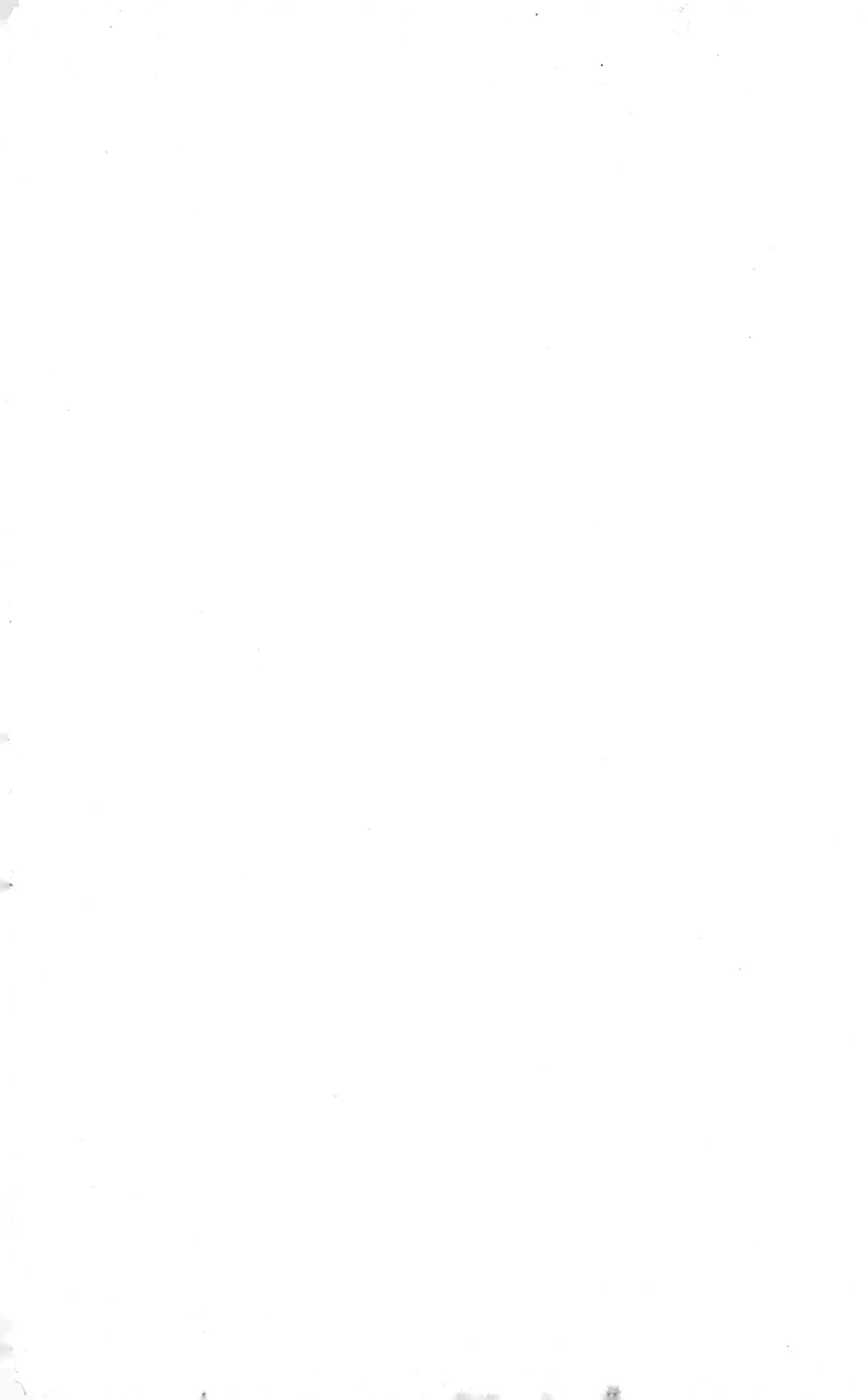